Advanced Neurosurgical Technologies:

Multidisciplinary Collaboration, Implementation, and Barriers

Soobia Saeed
https://orcid.org/0000-0002-9026-6130
Taylor's University, Malaysia

Mohsin Qadeer
https://orcid.org/0000-0001-7509-6885
Ziauddin University, Pakistan

IGI Global
Scientific Publishing
Publishing Tomorrow's Research Today

Vice President of Editorial Melissa Wagner
Director of Acquisitions Mikaela Felty
Director of Book Development Jocelynn Hessler
Production Manager Mike Brehm
Cover Design Jose Rosado

Published in the United States of America by
IGI Global Scientific Publishing
701 East Chocolate Avenue
Hershey, PA, 17033, USA
Tel: 717-533-8845 | Fax: 717-533-7115
Website: https://www.igi-global.com E-mail: cust@igi-global.com

Library of Congress Cataloging-in-Publication Data

LCCN: 2025052865 (CIP Data Pending)
ISBN13: 9798337362342
Isbn13Softcover: 9798337362359
EISBN13: 9798337362366

British Cataloguing in Publication Data
A Cataloguing in Publication record for this book is available from the British Library.

Editors dedicated this book to their respective Families and colleagues.

Editorial Advisory Board

Table of Contents

Detailed Table of Contents

In orthopedic and neurosurgical research, bone regeneration has become a growing area of research as a result of continued innovation in stem cell–enhanced scaffolding and bioprinting technologies in recent years. Bone has the ability to regenerate naturally, however, large defects from trauma, tumors, or musculoskeletal disease continue to pose clinical challenges. We present multiple strategies for bone tissue engineering with a focus on the roles of mesenchymal stem cells (MSCs), bioinks, and scaffold-based regenerative methods. Newer innovations in 3D bioprinting approaches have allowed for development of biomimetic scaffolds with cellular differentiation, vascularization, and structural properties. Emphasis is placed on the implications of synthetic polymers, bioactive molecules, and exogenous signals on enhancing osteogenic potential and scaffold capabilities. Finally, artificial intelligence has made its way into imaging and scaffold and regenerative design, creating an opportunity to rethink scaffold approach and maximize the potential outcomes of bone repair.

Lumbar disc prolapses (LDP), commonly known as herniated or slipped discs, is responsible for lower back pain and radiculopathy worldwide. The ongoing institutional audit and literature review is the one that the authors rely on to evaluate management strategies for lumbar disc prolapse through hospital-based records (n = 70) in addition to previously published studies for the sake of contextual comparison. The results of the study characterize treatment trends and outcomes but do not provide direct statistical comparisons as the authors did not standardize medication protocols across cases. Conservative treatments—e.g., analgesics, anti-inflammatories, muscle relaxants, neurotrophic supplementation, physiotherapy, etc.—are the first choice of treatment, showing sufficient symptom relief, functional recovery, and stable clinical outcomes. Surgery, especially microdiscectomy is done in cases with persistent neurologic deficits or pain despite conservative treatment, providing superior short-term relief but with similar long-term outcomes to conservative care.

This chapter explores the transformative role of emerging technologies in cranial and spine surgery, focusing on AI, Neuronavigation, Intraoperative Imaging, Augmented Reality (AR), 3D Printing, and Robotic-Assisted Systems. These tools are revolutionizing surgical precision, reducing invasiveness, and improving patient outcomes across all stages of care. Real-world case studies demonstrate measurable improvements in accuracy, recovery, and safety. The chapter also examines key challenges, including high costs, regulatory hurdles, limited training, and ethical concerns such as data privacy and algorithmic transparency. It emphasizes the need for multidisciplinary collaboration among neurosurgeons, engineers, data scientists, and policymakers to ensure equitable and successful adoption. Additionally, the chapter outlines future research directions aimed at closing access gaps, enhancing AI integration, and establishing ethical frameworks for responsible technology use. It provides a comprehensive guide for advancing neurosurgical practice through innovation.

The convergence of artificial intelligence (AI) and neurosurgery has transformed diagnostic precision, preoperative planning, and postoperative monitoring through the integration of advanced data analytics and imaging technologies. However, the centralized storage of sensitive medical data poses significant challenges to patient privacy and data protection, particularly within neurosurgical domains that rely heavily on neuroimaging and electrophysiological datasets. This study explores the implementation of federated learning (FL) as a privacy-preserving approach for AI-driven disease prediction in neurosurgical technologies. The proposed MediPro system integrates convolutional neural networks (CNNs) with federated learning and encrypted communication protocols to analyze MRI and CT scans, offering real-time, AI-assisted preliminary diagnosis while adhering to regulatory standards such as the Personal Data Protection Act (PDPA)

The chapter presents cutting-edge surgical advances, neuronavigation, intraoperative MRI (iMRI), and 5-aminolevulinic acid (5-ALA) fluorescence-guided resection techniques for treating complex intracranial tumors and their implications for clinical care. These advances allow the surgeon to visualize the tumor in real time and know where the tumor begins and ends—all of which improve surgical accuracy, decrease complications and increase extents of resection (EOR). Neuronavigation, often described as a "GPS for the brain," uses data from multiple imaging modalities (CT, MRI, and functional studies) to develop an intraoperative 3D map of the intraoperative anatomy. This increases surgical finesse, reduces the injury to normal brain, and promotes more aggressive tumor resection. The development of neuronavigation has changed from the initial stereotactic frame, to incorporating a frameless intraoperative mapping approach to now being image-integrated (providing dynamic image updates)—and provides an important opportunity to improve surgical precision.

Brain tumors are a major health problem and the only way to improve the outcome of the patients is to diagnose them accurately and very quickly. MRI scanning is usually the manual method of interpreting which suffers from being slow and varying between radiologists. In this research, a totally new AI method has been proposed that relies mostly on the Convolutional Neural Network (CNN) techniques for brain tumor classification. The model has been prepared and assessed using the Brain Tumor MRI Dataset, which is publicly available, and it covers four different tumor types: glioma, meningioma, pituitary tumor, and no tumor. As part of data preprocessing, normalization, augmentation, and image resizing were performed in order to increase the model's robustness and generalization. The CNN setup was made to automatically pick out the spatial features and appropriate patterns that are linked to tumor identification thus eliminating the manual feature engineering process.

The introduction of robotic surgical technology for instrumentation in spinal surgery is a breakthrough of tremendous importance to spinal surgical practice in terms of precision, safety, workflow, and efficiency. Robotic assisted systems utilize a targeting device that supports the placement of pedicle screws to within one millimeter of perceived accuracy while allowing for less intra-operative radiation exposure and decreased soft tissue trauma. Specifically, studies comparing robotic assisted techniques and workflow to traditional freehand or fluoroscopy guided techniques have demonstrated improved targeted accuracy, and fewer pedicle screw breaches with performance of greater than 90% and even >96% with some robotic systems. Briefly, the accuracy of several robotic platforms for the placement of pedicle screws, including Medtronic's Mazor X; Globus Medical's ExcelsiusGPS; and Brainlab's Cirq, have been evaluated to demonstrate accuracy >96%.

A brain stroke is a very serious health issue that is responsible for about 10% of death cases all over the world (nearly 6 million people) in 2019, and it is one of the top 10 causes of death and long-term disability in many countries. The medical community tries to turn this around by focusing on early diagnosis and treatment. Usually, other methods may not be available in developing regions where diagnosis and treatment are done using primitive tools. This project aims to employ the ever-increasing electronic health records together with data science to develop a predictive model that will detect high-risk individuals over stroke based on their health and lifestyle factors. The research is based on the Brain Stroke Dataset from Kaggle, which contains 4981 records with 11 attributes, including age, hypertension, heart disease, and smoking habits as the most important ones.

Foreword

The era of precision, personalization, and patient-centered care has brought about a huge change in the role of CT imaging, which is now not only the mainstay of diagnostics but also the most significant player in personalized surgical planning and implant design. This book is exactly at the right time when artificial intelligence, 3-D printing, and individual treatment protocols are changing the very criteria of surgical excellence. By looking at the optimization of CT parameters—voxel size, slice thickness, matrix resolution, and reconstruction algorithms—it helps clinicians, biomedical engineers, and researchers to break through the barriers that have existed for a long time in terms of accuracy in manipulation-based interventions.

What makes this book different is its very strong emphasis on the real-world application of the techniques, particularly in neurosurgery and orthopedic surgery. The combination of basic principles, advanced image-processing techniques, and case-based applications gives a complete resource for both seasoned professionals and novice researchers. Moreover, the book's discussion of AI-augmented analytics and 3D printing underlines the cross-disciplinary collaboration that is driving the future of personalized medicine.

My warmest congratulations are offered to Dr. Mohsin Qadeer and Dr. Soobia Saeed for their foresight and hard work in uniting the world's specialists to participate in this important project. Their editorial direction guarantees that the book will not only be a tough academic reference but also a useful guide for improving accuracy in clinical practice.

The viewers will find this work an indispensable help in their journey to innovation and patient outcome enhancement, as the health care sector continues its transition towards personalized, evidence-based decision-making.

Muhammad Riaz

University of Colorado, USA & Denver Health Medical Center, Children's Hospital Colorado, USA

Preface

Neurosurgery is an area of medicine that is experiencing great changes due to the combination of different technologies. The advanced imaging, minimally invasive techniques, intelligent computational systems, biologics, robotics, and precision-based surgical workflows are the main driving forces behind the changes. The complexity of brain and spine diseases is one of the factors that boost the demand for tools to improve accuracy, minimize complications, and customize treatment. The book, Multidisciplinary Collaboration and Implementation Barriers in Advanced Neurosurgical Technologies, discusses the role of the most advanced technologies in the regeneration of the neurosurgery field and the new standards for patient care. The different contributing authors present a thorough and multifaceted perspective on the technologies' implementation, the barriers to their adoption, and the cooperation models that are essential for the success of innovations in practical clinical settings.

OVERVIEW OF THE SUBJECT MATTER

At present, the neurosurgery field is one of the most advanced and interdisciplinary areas of medicine, as it combines technology, biomedical engineering, computational science, and the clinical acumen of experienced surgeons. The use of such tools as neuronavigation systems, computerized imaging during surgery, 3-D printing, augmented reality, AI-assisted diagnosis, robotics for spine surgeries, and biological implants has pushed the boundaries of the surgical possibilities to a great extent. Nevertheless, the challenges faced are still very significant, such as integration of new technologies into existing processes, approval of new methods and tools by the regulatory bodies, high costs, lack of trained personnel, incompatibility among different systems, and variability among patients.

The goal of this book is to give the reader a well-organized and comprehensive insight into the new technologies that will be coming up, with the emphasis being on their use in clinics, the technical basis, and the barriers to their acceptance in day-to-day practice. The basic idea is that neurosurgical innovations cannot prosper on their own; instead, they depend on the regular exchange of ideas and the collaboration of different medical professionals including neurosurgeons, biomedical engineers, radiologists, computer scientists, AI experts, neuroscientists, anesthesiologists, rehabilitation specialists, and even the global regulatory authorities.

The Topic's Relevance in Today's World

Across the globe, healthcare systems are moving towards precision medicine—personalized treatment that is highly dependent on data and is further supported by imaging and computational intelligence. Neurosurgery, being one of the most difficult specialties in terms of technique, is leading the way in this change. The present-day neurosurgery scenario is influenced by:

- An uptick in brain tumors, degenerative spinal diseases, trauma, and blood vessel disorders.
- Patients' higher expectations regarding less invasive, image-guided procedures that come with quicker recovery times.
- Incorporation of AI and machine learning into diagnosis, planning of surgery, and forecasting of results.
- A worldwide collaboration working on the unifying of surgical workflows and making cutting-edge technology more widely accessible.
- Patient-specific implants and anatomical models are made possible through additive manufacturing and 3-D printing.

Target Audience

This volume targets a wide range of multidisciplinary readers, such as:

- Neurosurgeons and residents in neurosurgery
- Surgeons specializing in spinal surgery and orthopedic surgery

- Professionals involved in the development of medical devices and biomedical engineering
- Radiologists and specialists in neuroradiology
- Artificial intelligence and machine learning researchers who focus on the healthcare sector
- Developers of robotics and augmented reality
- Experts in surgical planning and navigation
- Clinical researchers and researchers in academia
- Policymakers, regulators, and healthcare administrators
- Students and junior scientists are starting their research in neurosurgical technology

The book by considering both the clinical and engineering viewpoints, thus it is the one to effectively link together the worlds of innovation and implementation, therefore, its being academic, clinical and industrial audiences' necessities.

CHAPTER-BY-CHAPTER DESCRIPTION

Chapter 1. Bone Regeneration Strategies: Stem Cell-Enhanced Scaffold and Bioprinting in Neurosurgery

In orthopedic and neurosurgical research, bone regeneration has become a growing area of research as a result of continued innovation in stem cell–enhanced scaffolding and bioprinting technologies in recent years. Bone has the ability to regenerate naturally, however, large defects from trauma, tumors, or musculoskeletal disease continue to pose clinical challenges. We present multiple strategies for bone tissue engineering with a focus on the roles of mesenchymal stem cells (MSCs), bioinks, and scaffold-based regenerative methods. Newer innovations in 3D bioprinting approaches have allowed for development of biomimetic scaffolds with cellular differentiation, vascularization, and structural properties. Emphasis is placed on the implications of synthetic polymers, bioactive molecules, and exogenous signals on enhancing osteogenic potential and scaffold capabilities. Finally, artificial intelligence has made its way into imaging and scaffold and regenerative design, creating an opportunity to rethink scaffold approach and maximize the potential outcomes of bone repair.

Chapter 2. Institutional Audit for Clinical Outcomes and Management Strategies in Lumbar Disc Prolapse: A Comprehensive Review of Patient Recovery and Surgical Interventions

Lumbar disc prolapses (LDP), commonly known as herniated or slipped discs, is responsible for lower back pain and radiculopathy worldwide. The ongoing institutional audit and literature review is the one that the authors rely on to evaluate management strategies for lumbar disc prolapse through hospital-based records (n = 70) in addition to previously published studies for the sake of contextual comparison. The results of the study characterize treatment trends and outcomes but do not provide direct statistical comparisons as the authors did not standardize medication protocols across cases. Conservative treatments—e.g., analgesics, anti-inflammatories, muscle relaxants, neurotrophic supplementation, physiotherapy, etc.—are the first choice of treatment, showing sufficient symptom relief, functional recovery, and stable clinical outcomes. Surgery, especially microdiscectomy is done in cases with persistent neurologic deficits or pain despite conservative treatment, providing superior short-term relief but with similar long-term outcomes to conservative care.

Chapter 3. Transformative Technologies in Cranial and Spine Surgery: From AI Integration to Clinical Implementation

This chapter explores the transformative role of emerging technologies in cranial and spine surgery, focusing on AI, Neuronavigation, Intraoperative Imaging, Augmented Reality (AR), 3D Printing, and Robotic-Assisted Systems. These tools are revolutionizing surgical precision, reducing invasiveness, and improving patient outcomes across all stages of care. Real-world case studies demonstrate measurable improvements in accuracy, recovery, and safety. The chapter also examines key challenges, including high costs, regulatory hurdles, limited training, and ethical concerns such as data privacy and algorithmic transparency. It emphasizes the need for multidisciplinary collaboration among neurosurgeons, engineers, data scientists, and policymakers to ensure equitable and successful adoption. Additionally, the chapter outlines future research directions aimed at closing access gaps, enhancing AI integration, and establishing ethical frameworks for responsible technology use. It provides a comprehensive guide for advancing neurosurgical practice through innovation.

Chapter 4. AI-Driven Disease Prediction Through Federated Learning: Privacy-Preserving Innovations in Neurosurgical Technologies

The convergence of artificial intelligence (AI) and neurosurgery has transformed diagnostic precision, preoperative planning, and postoperative monitoring through the integration of advanced data analytics and imaging technologies. However, the centralized storage of sensitive medical data poses significant challenges to patient privacy and data protection, particularly within neurosurgical domains that rely heavily on neuroimaging and electrophysiological datasets. This study explores the implementation of federated learning (FL) as a privacy-preserving approach for AI-driven disease prediction in neurosurgical technologies. The proposed MediPro system integrates convolutional neural networks (CNNs) with federated learning and encrypted communication protocols to analyze MRI and CT scans, offering real-time, AI-assisted preliminary diagnosis while adhering to regulatory standards such as the Personal Data Protection Act (PDPA)

Chapter 5. Implementation of Neuronavigation-Guided Resection in Complex Intracranial Tumors

The chapter presents cutting-edge surgical advances, neuronavigation, intraoperative MRI (iMRI), and 5-aminolevulinic acid (5-ALA) fluorescence-guided resection techniques for treating complex intracranial tumors and their implications for clinical care. These advances allow the surgeon to visualize the tumor in real time and know where the tumor begins and ends—all of which improve surgical accuracy, decrease complications and increase extents of resection (EOR). Neuronavigation, often described as a "GPS for the brain," uses data from multiple imaging modalities (CT, MRI, and functional studies) to develop an intraoperative 3D map of the intraoperative anatomy.

This increases surgical finesse, reduces the injury to normal brain, and promotes more aggressive tumor resection. The development of neuronavigation has changed from the initial stereotactic frame, to incorporating a frameless intraoperative mapping approach to now being image-integrated (providing dynamic image updates)—and provides an important opportunity to improve surgical precision.

Chapter 6. Automated Brain Tumor Classification from MRI Images Using Convolutional Neural Networks An AI-Driven Diagnostic Approach

Brain tumors are a major health problem and the only way to improve the outcome of the patients is to diagnose them accurately and very quickly. MRI scanning is usually the manual method of interpreting which suffers from being slow and varying between radiologists. In this research, a totally new AI method has been proposed that relies mostly on the Convolutional Neural Network (CNN) techniques for brain tumor classification. The model has been prepared and assessed using the Brain Tumor MRI Dataset, which is publicly available, and it covers four different tumor types: glioma, meningioma, pituitary tumor, and no tumor. As part of data preprocessing, normalization, augmentation, and image resizing were performed in order to increase the model's robustness and generalization. The CNN setup was made to automatically pick out the spatial features and appropriate patterns that are linked to tumor identification thus eliminating the manual feature engineering process.

Chapter 7. Surgical Robotics in Spine Instrumentation: Real-World Applications, Challenges, and the Role of Medical Education

The introduction of robotic surgical technology for instrumentation in spinal surgery is a breakthrough of tremendous importance to spinal surgical practice in terms of precision, safety, workflow, and efficiency. Robotic assisted systems utilize a targeting device that supports the placement of pedicle screws to within one millimeter of perceived accuracy while allowing for less intra-operative radiation exposure and decreased soft tissue trauma. Specifically, studies comparing robotic assisted techniques and workflow to traditional freehand or fluoroscopy guided techniques have demonstrated improved targeted accuracy, and fewer pedicle screw breaches with performance of greater than 90% and even >96% with some robotic systems. Briefly, the accuracy of several robotic platforms for the placement of pedicle screws, including Medtronic's Mazor X; Globus Medical's ExcelsiusGPS; and Brainlab's Cirq, have been evaluated to demonstrate accuracy >96%.

Chapter 8. Data-Driven Prediction of Brain Stroke Risk Using Machine Learning Techniques on Healthcare

A brain stroke is a very serious health issue that is responsible for about 10% of death cases all over the world (nearly 6 million people) in 2019, and it is one of the top 10 causes of death and long-term disability in many countries. The medical community tries to turn this around by focusing on early diagnosis and treatment. Usually, other methods may not be available in developing regions where diagnosis and treatment are done using primitive tools. This project aims to employ the ever-increasing electronic health records together with data science to develop a predictive model that will detect high-risk individuals over stroke based on their health and lifestyle factors. The research is based on the Brain Stroke Dataset from Kaggle, which contains 4981 records with 11 attributes, including age, hypertension, heart disease, and smoking habits as the most important ones.

Chapter 9. Implementation of Augmented Reality in Cranial Trauma Reconstruction

Cranial trauma involving patients with depressed skull fractures and complex craniofacial injuries has not lost its status of very difficult surgical operations among neurosurgery and reconstruction. In spite of the introduction of sophisticated imaging and 3D printing, the intra-operative accuracy and anatomical fidelity challenge is still existing. The paper discusses the introduction of Augmented Reality (AR) in the field of cranial trauma reconstruction and points out the uses of AR in surgical visualization, precision implant, and workflow efficiency. Clinical trials, technical reports, and experimental studies on AR with 3D-printed PEEK implants, neuronavigation, and AI-assisted modeling were systematically collected from the Google Scholar database over a period of five years from 2019 to 2025.

Chapter 10. Real-Time Neurophysiological Monitoring during Scoliosis Correction Surgeries

Complex deformity treatment involves the mechanical, vascular, and neurological strain, there is a significant risk of iatrogenic spinal cord or nerve injury during scoliosis correction surgery. One essential tool for improving surgical safety and accuracy is real-time intraoperative neurophysiological monitoring, or RT-IONM. The concepts, processes, and data pertaining to RT-IONM during scoliosis correction surgeries are thoroughly reviewed in this chapter. The major goal of a systematic review and meta-analysis is to show that IONM is linked to less neurological sequelae following surgery; however, because of research heterogeneity and a lack of randomized data, the overall quality of the evidence is still moderate. Further evidence that multimodal IONM—combining motor evoked potentials (MEPs), somatosensory evoked potentials (SSEPs), and electromyography (EMG)—increases sensitivity and predictive value, especially in high-risk deformity cases, comes from scoliosis-specific data from recent multicenter studies, such as the Scoliosis Research Society database (2013–2023).

Acknowledgment

We would like to extend our heartfelt appreciation to all those who contributed to the successful completion of this project. This endeavor would not have been possible without the collective support and collaboration of many individuals.

First and foremost, we owe sincere thanks to all authors who shared their knowledge, insights, and experience in their chapter contributions. They were ardent supporters of this project and so observed the time limits for the various stages with great discipline, without which this book could never have reached completion.

We are also eternally grateful for the reviewers' excellent work. Their thoughtful and constructive comments greatly improved the chapters' quality, clarity, and coherence. Many of the authors were also reviewers, to whom we extend especial thanks for their commitment and time

Of course, a last but not least, profound thanks are due to our families and friends for their endless support, love, prayers, and understanding. Their encouragement and sacrifices were paramount for our timely completion of this project.

Soobia Saeed

Taylor's University, Malaysia

Mohsin Qadeer

National Medical Center, Pakistan

Chapter 1
Bone Regeneration Strategies:
Stem Cell-Enhanced Scaffold and Bioprinting in Neurosurgery

Rubina Ghani
https://orcid.org/0000-0003-1923-7924
Sohail University, Pakistan

Zeelaf A. Shahid
https://orcid.org/0000-0002-5396-4503
Jinnah Medical and Dental College, Pakistan

ABSTRACT

In orthopedic and neurosurgical research, bone regeneration has become a growing area of research as a result of continued innovation in stem cell–enhanced scaffolding and bioprinting technologies in recent years. Bone has the ability to regenerate naturally, however, large defects from trauma, tumors, or musculoskeletal disease continue to pose clinical challenges. We present multiple strategies for bone tissue engineering with a focus on the roles of mesenchymal stem cells (MSCs), bioinks, and scaffold-based regenerative methods. Newer innovations in 3D bioprinting approaches have allowed for development of biomimetic scaffolds with cellular differentiation, vascularization, and structural properties. Emphasis is placed on the implications of synthetic polymers, bioactive molecules, and exogenous signals on enhancing osteogenic potential and scaffold capabilities. Finally, artificial intelligence

DOI: 10.4018/979-8-3373-6234-2.ch001

has made its way into imaging and scaffold and regenerative design, creating an opportunity to rethink scaffold approach and maximize the potential outcomes of bone repair.

1. INTRODUCTION

Bone has an extraordinary ability for self-repair. The employment of stem cells with the capacity for self-repair and regeneration as a way to replace damaged and diseased tissues and organs represents new therapeutic possibilities for conventional intractable conditions. Of the few organs with regenerative capacity, bone is a dynamic connective tissue with a complex cellular makeup characterized by a highly specialized organic–inorganic structure (Perez et al., 2018). Thus, tissues engineering and cell-based tissue engineering have become novel approaches to fracture and bone defect management. Bone has many important biological functions: providing mobility for the body, supporting the internal organs, ensuring hematopoietic cells, and acting as a critical mineral store (Iaquinta et al., 2019).

The dilemma for musculoskeletal surgeons is healing huge bony defects. Segmental bone defects from trauma, tumors, or other musculoskeletal problems affect millions per year in the loss of quality of life. Bone tissue is known to be able to remodel well when the defect is small, but it is unable to degenerate across segmental and larger gaps without intervention. Thus, grafting materials are often resorted to, and autologous bone grafts are still the gold standard for treating major bony defects.

Regrettably, classical regenerative medicine works with stem cell suspensions face a series of problems such as cell deaths and sub-optimal grafting results. Concerns also linger over the usage of biomaterial and/or enzymatic agents (trypsin) such as in passaging the stem cells, while they might also pass adverse effects on stem cell viability and functionality which would eventually hamper the repair and regenerative potential.

The use of enzyme and biomaterials such as trypsin, during traditional two-dimensional (2D) cell culture processes often compromises the viability and function of cells, leading to reduced therapeutic potential of any transplanted cells at the target site. Three-dimensional (3D) cell culture methods are becoming more popular and more of a focus, because they may provide a better approximation of native biological environments in which cells can experience pertinent cell–cell and cell–extracellular matrix (ECM) interactions. These methods consistently present favorable outcomes in various disease models (P et al., 2018; Ke-Chunu et al., 2024). In general, these methods make use of scaffolds made from biocompatible and often biodegradable materials as carriers for stem cells. However, the use of exogenous biomaterials in cell and scaffold composites raises questions about the possible immune response and biosafety issues with biomechanical stability and degradation of scaffold materials (Zhang et al., 2021). Bone regenerative therapy (BRT) is one of the most successful stem cell-based strategies, which consists of a synergistic approach using both mesenchymal progenitor cells with osteogenic potential, bioactive factors that prime osteogenic differentiation, and multiple biocompatible scaffold materials. The underlying basis of BRT is to use cell friendly biomaterials as scaffolds for the repair of large bone defect sites. This article offers an extensive, cutting-edge overview of scaffold-based strategies in bone tissue engineering. It identifies important challenges and barriers, outlines recent developments and uses, and identifies possible directions for the future.

The main types of stem cell used for bone regeneration are bone marrow-derived mesenchymal stem cells (BMSCs), mesenchymal stem cells obtained from the oral cavity, and adipose stem cells (ASCs). Cells derived from the umbilical vein and endothelial progenitor cells are utilized for neovascularization. The use of stem cells for tissue engineering with a scaffold is more effective than using the scaffold alone for bone regeneration, regardless of the type of stem cell. Although there are several types of scaffolds tested in preclinical studies, composite biomaterials represent an effective type of scaffold. Preclinical studies evaluating the use of cells and scaffolds for bone regeneration have primarily used bioceramic scaffolds (especially β-tricalcium phosphate (β-TCP) and biodegradable polymers that are both osteoconductive and biocompatible.

Bone grafts from an autologous source, allograft options, and alternative biomaterials have been utilized for reconstruction of large bone defects. Autologous grafts, in particular, have the advantage of presenting the best osteogenic potential, possess adequate mechanical strength, and do not have a risk of viral transmission or immunogenicity. However, autologous grafts do have certain limitations due to available autologous bone quantity and complications from the harvest site, including morbidity, hematoma, or nerve injury (Ebraheim et al., 2000; Myeroff & Archdeacon, 2011).

Allografts provide immediate osteoconduction and mechanical stability after surgery with no supply limitations. Masaoka et al. (2016) showed the simplicity of a composite of β-tricalcium phosphate (β-TCP) with monkey bone marrow mesenchymal stem cells (MSCs) for repair of large defects in a model with non-human primates.

Although these innovations have occurred, high complication rates exist with large intercalary grafts, especially for osseous neoplasms or adjuvant therapy. As a solution, synthetic calcium phosphate-based substitutes have been introduced into clinical practice, specifically hydroxyapatite and/or tricalcium phosphate (TCP) graft materials. These substitutes reduce the concerns of viral transmission and limited supply. While modifications to these materials have led to some improvements in their osteogenic properties, they have not achieved enough of an improvement to completely regenerate large segmental defects.

2. THE SOURCES OF STEM CELLS

The biological properties and therapeutic use of stem cells are key factors in selecting stem cells for tissue engineering. Generally, stem cells can be broadly classified as pluripotent or adult stem cells. Pluripotent stem cells, such as embryonic stem cells (ESCs), can potentially differentiate to form the majority of cell types. Despite exploring a variety of applications for ESCs' potential for heterogeneous differentiation, immunological rejection, mutation susceptibility (high mutation rates), and ethical concerns have all limited their use in clinical settings.

Induced pluripotent stem cells (iPSCs) are obtained through the reprogramming of adult somatic cells. iPSCs possess the ability to develop into a variety of cell types such as cardiomyocytes, neurons, hepatocytes, and endothelial cells, which signifies their importance in regenerative medicine, disease modeling, and drug development, although they also present major clinical challenges such as immune response, genetic instability, and tumor formation (Newsome et al., 2018). Hematopoietic stem cells (HSCs) are precursors to myeloid and lymphoid lineages and have shown some therapeutic capability in the clinic, namely in the case of liver regeneration using hepatic progenitor cells (Spahr et al., 2013; Siapati et al., 2022). Neural stem cells (NSCs) are capable of differentiating into neurons, oligodendrocytes, and astrocytes and are thought to be involved in repairs and neurogenesis through social interactions promoted by their activity in the nervous system (Gage et al., 2000). For example, they may play a neuroprotective role by releasing glial cell line-derived neurotrophic factor (GDNF).

Mesenchymal stem cells (MSCs) are a very flexible cell type in regenerative medicine and have the potential to be used in various ways. They can be isolated from different tissues such as bone marrow, fat, dental pulp, periodontal ligaments, umbilical cord, and placenta. The two main sources of MSCs that are most commonly used are adipose-derived stem cells (ADSCs) and bone marrow-derived MSCs (BMMSCs). One of the major sources of factors that stimulate the growth and formation of blood vessels is MSCs and among these factors are vascular endothelial growth factor (VEGF) and hepatocyte growth factor (HGF)(Ke-Chun et al., 2024). In addition to this, MSCs can interact with various types of immune cells, such as T cells, B cells, and natural killer (NK) cells, and by that, they could possibly alter the immune system through the signaling of several immune-mediated cytokines like interleukin 10 (IL-10), prostaglandin E2 (PGE2), transforming growth factor-beta (TGF-β), indoleamine 2,3-dioxygenase (IDO), and nitric oxide (Gao et al., 2016).

Bone tissue engineering (BTE) has surfaced as an exciting, interdisciplinary area within regenerative medicine that is focused on developing biomaterials of great utility, incorporating biomimetic scaffolds for bone repair and regeneration. Taken together the biological characteristics in conjunction with the materials and engineering aspects of the field, BTE systems aim to overcome the constraints of bone repair techniques utilized in the clinic today (i.e. autografts and allografts). There have been a number of recent developments in BTE systems with the intent to engineer dynamic, bioresponsive scaffolds that replicate the structure and function of the natural extracellular matrix (ECM) to make substantial advances in restoring the structural integrity and function of bone tissue.

Considered to be the biggest breakthrough in regenerative medicine would be the development of newer intelligent scaffold systems integrating bioactive materials with a responsive element allowing real-time adaptations. This field has seen huge breakthroughs of late, with studies giving examples of scaffold designs that change their mechanical and biochemical properties dynamically for the best tissue regeneration.

The process of bone formation, or ossification (also called osteogenesis), commences between the sixth and seventh weeks of embryonic development. This remarkable process specifically involves Mesenchymal Stem Cells (MSCs), multi-potent progenitor cells found in the bone marrow and various other tissues. MSCs can differentiate into many types of cells, such as osteogenic lineage (shown in Figure 1). Four main cellular types are significant in the process of bone development, and each cell type has its own unique functional role in the life cycle and structural integrity of bone.

Osteogenic cells (osteoprogenitor cells), located primarily in the periosteum and endosteum (significant sites of growth and repair), are the progenitor cells in the osteoblastic lineage of differentiation. These progenitor cells will become osteoblasts that perform their primary role in the process of bone development by creating an amorphous matrix that will later mineralize into osteoid, the unmineralized matrix of bone. Osteoid will later become mineralized by the deposition of calcium phosphate crystals providing structural stability to bone. Once the osteoblast has laid down sufficient matrix, they become trapped within the bone and differentiate to become osteocytes - cells that serve to regulate bone homeostasis and signaling (Kenkre & Bassett, 2018; Einhorn et al. 2004).

Figure 1. It shows the structure of a typical long bone.

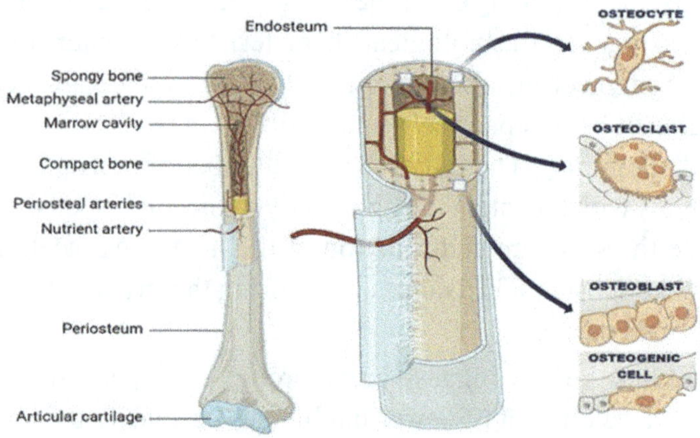

3. BONE REMODELING

Bone is a tissue with high metabolic activity that continuously remodels in a cyclical model that is vital for the mechanical competence of the skeleton and metabolic functions in vertebrates. The remodeling cycle includes five distinct phases of remodeling shown in Figure 2: activation, resorption, reversal, formation, and termination. These remodeling phases represent discrete cellular and biochemical processes that tailor the rate of bone resorption and formation of new bone. Initiation of the remodeling process begins with the activation phase, which occurs when bone-lining cells migrate away from the adjacent bone surface to create a raised canopy over the area selected for resorption. This process is initiated by a tightly regulated sequence that leads to coordination of the bone maintenance and renewal processes.

Figure 2. shows the different stages of bone remodeling.

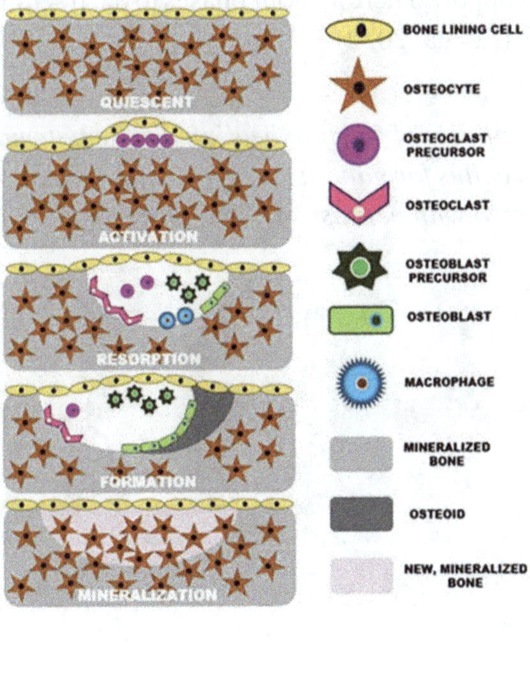

4. BONE REPAIR

Bone healing can occur through either a primary or a secondary mechanism, depending on the type of fracture and the degree of damage. Primary bone healing occurs when the gap in the fracture is small (less than 0.1 mm), and if there is enough stabilization, the fracture will ossify directly with no visible callus formation (Wang et al., 2017). Primary bone healing is uncommon and generally requires surgical stabilization to obtain a rigid fixation and an anatomical alignment of the fracture ends. Secondary bone healing occurs when the gap is larger than 0.1 mm (but no larger than twice the diameter of the bone) (Ledda, 2022). A soft callus develops in the gap and matures until the original bone structure is restored.

Bone healing processes remain incompletely understood, although they will incorporate an adequate number of viable osteogenic cells, an adequate connective tissue matrix, adequate vascularity and growth factors, and adequate mechanical support. There are four phases to the fracture repair process, shown in Figure 3 (Ledda, 2022).

Figure 3. The four phases of fracture healing: (a) hematoma formation; (b) fibrocartilaginous callus formation; (c) bony callus formation; and (d) bone remodeling. (Adapted with permission from Biorender.com).

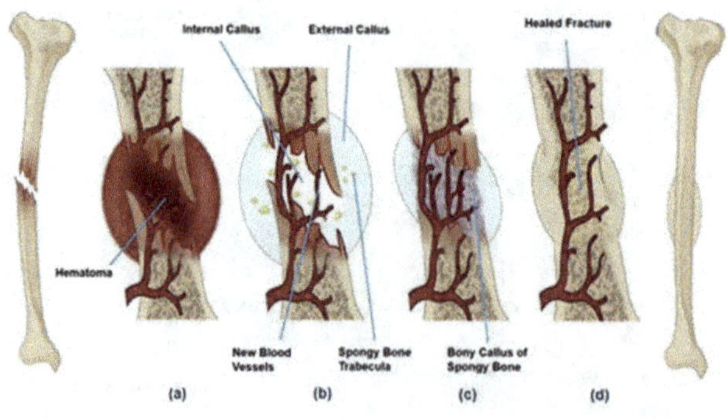

4.1 New Interventions: Spinal Cord Injury

Spinal Cord Injury (SCI) is a significant neurological condition that occurs through damage to the spine resulting in partial loss or total loss of motor and sensory function below the injury level. Recovery and rehabilitation form the focus of rehabilitation specialists and can be a lengthy and multi-faceted approach that involves new and established therapeutic options to optimize functional outcomes for people with SCI (Eckert & Martin, 2017). SCI are disabling because of the structural breakdown of neurons and axons in the spinal cord, and injuries can be represented predominantly through traumatic mechanisms. The primary injury begins as a physical mechanical injury to the neural tissues, resulting in a cascade of associated cellular and molecular events that lead to blood–spinal cord barrier disruption. Secondary injury involves a multitude of processes including but not limited to inflammation, excitotoxicity, and oxidative stress. These processes then continue the neuronal loss and further contribute to decreased neuronal ability, which also affects neural regeneration/repair, as seen in figure 4. (Alizadeh et al., 2019).

Figure 4. Pathophysiological progression of spinal cord injury.

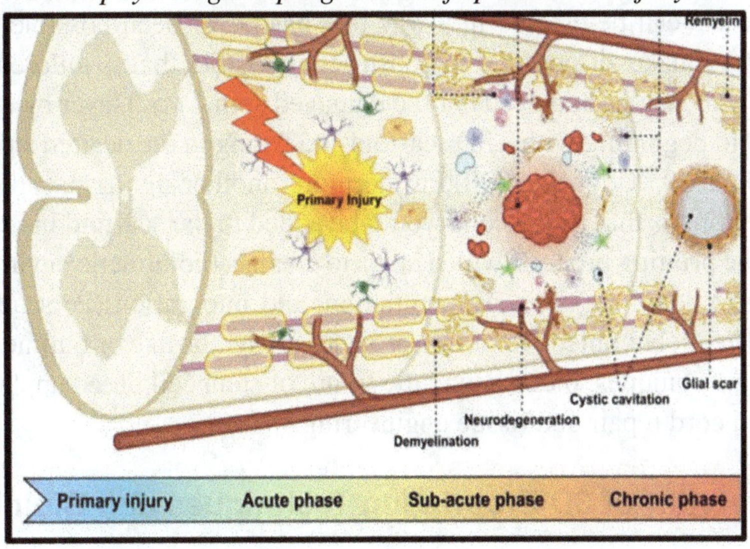

This Figure outlines the temporal sequence of the pathophysiological processes occurring following spinal cord injury (SCI) from injury to chronic stages. A novel approach to overcoming the drawbacks of earlier treatments for spinal cord injury (SCI) is tissue engineering (Jia & Li, 2024). In order to develop bioengineered structures that might support neural regeneration and function recovery, this highly interdisciplinary field integrates concepts from biology, engineering, and material science. Tissue engineering for

SCI will concentrate on bioengineered or synthetic scaffolds that replicate the extracellular matrix (ECM) environment in order to support neural cell survival, proliferation, and eventual differentiation (da Silva et al., 2023).

A novel approach to overcoming the drawbacks of earlier treatments for spinal cord injury (SCI) is tissue engineering (Jia & Li, 2024). In order to develop bioengineered structures that might support neural regeneration and function recovery, this highly interdisciplinary field integrates concepts from biology, engineering, and material science. Tissue engineering for SCI will concentrate on bioengineered or synthetic scaffolds that replicate the extracellular matrix (ECM) environment in order to support neural cell survival, proliferation, and eventual differentiation (da Silva et al., 2023).

A new stage of tissue engineering development, particularly for complex tissues like the spinal cord, has been triggered by the advent of 3D bioprinting (Saini et al., 2021). With the use of this technique, scaffolds with intricate geometric patterns and microarchitectures that closely resemble natural neural tissue can be created in a way that has never been possible before. Bioprinting makes it possible to construct a scaffold that is tailored to the specific dimensions and needs of the damaged spinal cord layer by layer, as opposed to beginning with a 3D scaffold and filling in the desired structures (Gu et al., 2020; Xie et al., 2020).Furthermore, another significant advantage of bioprinting is that living cells would be added to the scaffold in real-time during the printing process, which helps to create a biomimetic environment for improved cell survival, differentiation, and integration (Persaud et al., 2022). The global objective of this project will synthesize or outline 3D bioprinting techniques, bioinks, and the future of stem cell based applications for spinal cord repair and tissue engineering.

4.2 Overview of 3D Bioprinting Techniques and Bioinks

3D bioprinting has emerged as a revolutionary technology in repairing spinal cord injuries (SCI) serving as a means to engineer complex, biomimetic scaffolds for neuronal regeneration and re-establish functional neural circuits. Moreover, these scaffolds promote cell proliferation, and differentiation (Zarepour et al., 2021), induce the release of neurotrophic factors (Lu et al.,

2022; Jiu et al., 2024), and modulate inflammatory responses (Bedir et al., 2020; Szymoniuk et al., 2023, Ju et al., 2024).

There are four primary types of bioprinting which include: extrusion-based, inkjet-based, laser-assisted bioprinting, and stereolithography, each presenting certain advantages for scaffold fabrication (Yuan et al., 2022). Extrusion-based bioprinting is the most commonly used bioprinting which allows for the controlled deposition of bioinks with high viscosity and is therefore an efficient method of generating scaffold with appropriate mechanical stiffness (Gillispie et al., 2020). Inkjet-based bioprinting has the best spatial precision of the placement of cells and allows the systematic spatial distribution of cellular materials, but is restricted to low viscosity bioinks, which provide lower mechanical support (Kumar et al., 2020). Laser-assisted bioprinting has both greater resolution and cell viability but is less common due to cost and complexity (Ventura et al., 2021). Stereolithography employs vat polymerization for the generation of complex 3D geometries but can encounter challenges with photo-initiators causing possible cytotoxicity or lengthen print times (Kumar et al., 2020) (Figure 5).

Figure 5. Bioprinting techniques and applications in tissue engineering.

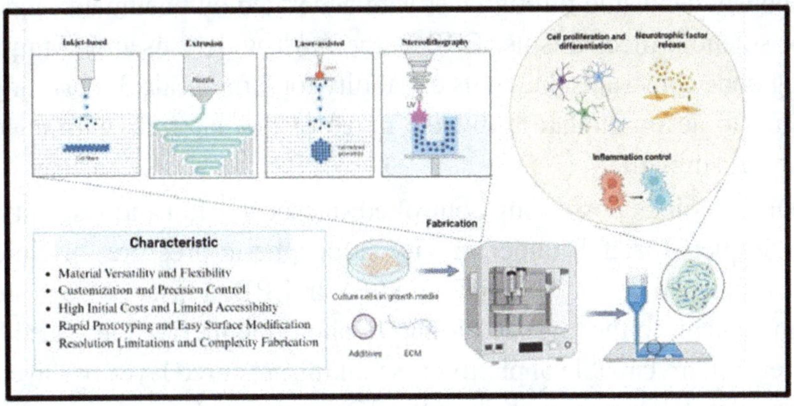

Typically, three common methods are employed in bone bioprinting, depending on the bioink used, including extrusion-based bioprinting (EBB), droplet-based bioprinting (DBB), and laser-based bioprinting (LBB). EBB disperses bioink from a syringe or nozzle to a build platform along a computer-aided design (CAD) of the desired target structure (see Figure 6A). Sites are filled with cylindrical filaments of materials deposited continuously via a stream supplied by a pneumatic, mechanical, or solenoid mechanism. EBB is the most commonly used method for bone constructs due to the ease of scaling to large 3D prints and the variety of biomaterials it can utilize with sufficient mechanical strength. On the right side of the figure, we see the post-fabrication phase, where the printed constructs are cultured in growth medium to enhance proliferation among other processes, differentiation, and secretion of neurotrophic factors as well as regulate inflammation. Regarding inflammation regulation, the red cells stand for M1 macrophages, which induce pro-inflammatory responses, while the blue cells stand for M2 macrophages that coordinate anti-inflammatory activity and tissue repair.

4.3 Bioprinting Apparatus

Three prevalent bioprinting methods are generally utilized in bone bioprinting, depending on the selected bioink formulation: extrusion-based bioprinting (EBB), droplet-based bioprinting (DBB), and laser-based bioprinting (LBB). EBB involves the extrusion of bioink from a syringe or nozzle onto the build platform, following a computer-aided design (CAD) model of the intended target structure (Figure 6A). Cylindrical filaments of material are continuously deposited through a stream generated by pneumatic, mechanical, or solenoid mechanisms. EBB is the most widely used technique for creating bone constructs due to its capability for large-scale 3D printing and its ability to accommodate a diverse range of biomaterials with adequate mechanical strength.

In DBB, bioinks possessing controlled surface tension and viscosity give rise to droplets that fall under gravity, atmospheric pressure, or fluid dynamics (Gudapati et al., 2019) (Figure 6B). In LBB, a laser pulse is steered through a mirror to the layer of bioink. In photopolymerization-based LBB, hydrogel systems capable of photo-crosslinking are cured layer-by-layer with an ultraviolet (UV) laser to produce the 3D construct of interest (Koch et al., 2019) (Figure 6C).

The most recent of all innovations, Aspiration-Assisted Bioprinting, allows one to manipulate and place cell spheroids with precision. It takes advantage of the formation of spheroids originating from various cell types at high density; using negative air pressure, it lifts these spheroids and deposits them on hydrogel substrates (Ayan et al., 2020) (Figure 6D). Often, these bioprinting techniques are integrated or hybridized to maximize the constructs' mechanical integrity and biological function.

Figure 6. Bioprinting technologies utilized for bone tissue include: (A) Extrusion-based bioprinting, which encompasses traditional pneumatic/piston extrusion (A1), coaxial nozzles designed for printing core–shell filaments (A2), dual-nozzle setups for bioprinting various bioinks (A3), and post-printing polymerization techniques for photocurable bioinks; (B) droplet-based bioprinting; (C) laser-based bioprinting; and (D) aspiration-assisted bioprinting.

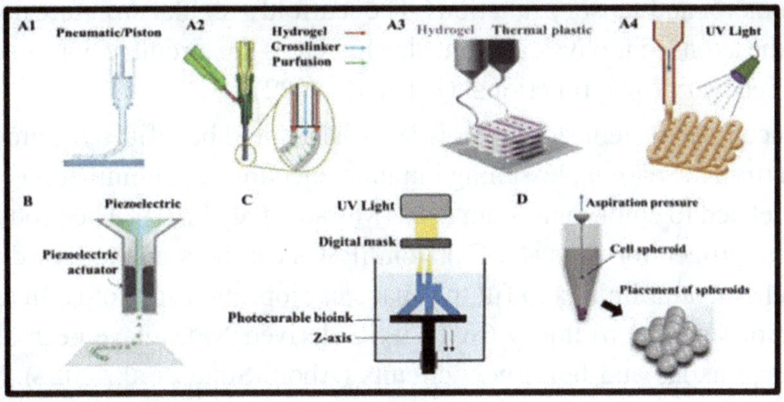

4.4 Role of Stem Cells in 3D Bioprinting for Spinal Cord Injury (SCI) Repair

Prominent in the 3D bioprinting process for the repair of spinal cord injury (SCI) is the role of stem cells, which hold the promise of replacing damaged neural tissue and restoring lost neurological function (Yuan et al., 2022). Neural stem cells are particularly useful in that they can differentiate into neurons, astrocytes, and oligodendrocytes, the primary cell types of the central nervous system (Ye et al., 2023Stem cell incorporation into the 3D bioprinting scaffolds most likely assists in their survival, proliferation, and even further direct differentiation right at the injury site. The use of NSCs, as well as induced pluripotent stem cell (iPSC)-derived progenitors and ectomesenchymal stem cells (EMSCs) has been reported through several studies in bioprinted constructs (Zarepour et al., 2021; Ju et al., 2024). Typically, these cells are encapsulated in hydrogels that replicate the extracellular matrix

(ECM) to create an appropriate microenvironment for their final maturation and integration with the host tissues (Lee et al., 2022).

The application of NSCs in 3D - bioprinted scaffolds has shown several promising results. With the scaffolds facilitating the process, axonal regeneration is boosted, glial scarring is suppressed, and SCI repair becomes a favorable option (Baker et al., 2019). Scaffolds with embedded NSCs can keep the cells alive and even allow them to differentiate at the site of lesion, which in turn, especially happens with the animal models of Liu et al., 2021, and Gao et al., 2024; Liu et al., 2022 who reported such significant changes in their motor and sensory functions. The scaffold's regular structure not only draws the axons to it physically but also recreates the circuitry that is needed for the recovery to be functional (Hu et al., 2022).

Induced pluripotent stem cells (iPSCs) also yield benefits by sources' selection from the patient, lessening immune rejection, and eliminating ethical issues related to embryonic stem cells (Moradi et al., 2019). The production of neural progenitor cells (NPCs) from iPSCs can be a method, or directly from other neural linings to fill the space in bioprinted scaffolds. In animal models of spinal cord injury (SCI), iPSC-derived NPCs have been able to regenerate axons and build new circuits (Aboul-Soud et al., 2021). When the cells are brought in with the help of 3D printed scaffolds, they exhibit improved integration with the surrounding tissues, better recovery of motor function, and less damage from secondary injury mechanisms, such as inflammation and glial scarring (Zheng et al., 2022).

Cranial neural crest-derived ectomesenchymal stem cells (EMSCs) represent a very good 3D bioprinting solution since these cells are able to differentiate into neurons and glial cells which are required for SCI repair. 3D bioprinting offers a high degree of precision in creating scaffolds that closely resemble the natural cell microenvironment, thus supporting cell growth and differentiation (Ma et al., 2022). Specific hydrogels can act as a scaffold while still allowing the structure to remain intact and gradually breaking down to release neurotrophic factors like brain-derived neurotrophic factor (BDNF), thereby aiding the development of functional neural tissue.

More recent research has demonstrated a progression of the field indicating that transplantation of human umbilical cord mesenchymal stem cells (MSCs) delivered on collagen/silk fibroin scaffolds, promote functional recovery from SCI. Next, a somewhat more recent methodology has focused on a 3D-printed collagen/silk fibroin scaffold infused with MSC-secretome (protein secreted from MSC) to act as a template for neural repair. The MSC-secretome, an ethically acceptable and stable alternative to MSC transplantation, is a combination of proteins secreted/metabolized by MSCs. The MSC-secretome has both shown to produce similar outcomes and promote nerve fiber regeneration, increased restoration of motor and similar functions, increased synaptic connections within the lesion area (Chen et al., 2022).

5. CHALLENGES AND FUTURE PERSPECTIVES

In spite of its promising potential in regenerative medicine, 3D printing application for spinal cord regeneration has multiple critical problems. Selecting and developing the appropriate bioinks as basic printable materials is a principal barrier. These bioinks should be biocompatible and should provide enough mechanical strength, rheology, and structural stability to support growth and integration of neural tissues. Nevertheless, many bioinks presently available are sourced from non-human systems, subjecting some immunogenic and infective potentialities. Furthermore, it remains exceedingly challenging to create materials that meet the complex mechano-biological-physicochemical requirements needed to stimulate spinal cord regeneration in an effective manner. In improving such capacity, further knowledge in biomaterial science, tissue engineering, and biofabrication techniques will be required, treating with the safe and functional integration within the host tissues.

6. FUTURE TRENDS IN 3D BIOPRINTING-BASED THERAPIES

With the advancement of 3D bioprinting of energy repairs, many treatment innovations are beginning to take shape that will significantly enhance treatment outcomes. One of the major advances discussed in Section 3 is incorporating sophisticated functional components within the bioprinted scaffolds. Future designs would fully incorporate conductive materials, bioactive molecules such as neurotrophic factors, therapeutic drugs, and stem cell-derived exosomes with designs that closely mimicked the architecture of the spinal cord microenvironment. This type of incorporation would positively influence the healing of the nervous system as well as the recovery of the functions concerned. One more major movement in the medical field is the progressively crucial role of personalized medicine, which can be traced back to the technological advancements in bioprinting, which are of utmost importance for creating scaffolds that are exactly fitting to a person's anatomical and pathological features. The customization of the scaffold guarantees a perfect fit to the injury that might, in the end, promote neural repair and functional recovery better than ever. All these trends combined denote a transition towards more precise, flexible, and effective regenerative solutions for SCI repair.

7. CONCLUSION

The development and renewal of bone tissue have benefited enormously from the combination of stem cell-based therapies and 3D bioprinting. It is now clear that biocompatible scaffolds, bioactive molecules, and stem cell implementations contribute to achieving the best results in bone healing and tissue integration. Although autologous bone grafts have typically set the standard for clinical procedures, drawbacks like morbidity at the harvesting site and limited supply have prompted studies into alternative biomaterials and tissue-engineered constructs.

Lately, the scaffold fabrication which closely resembles the extracellular matrix has been developed with the help of sophisticated bioprinting technologies, thus empowering the cellular processes of adhesion, proliferation, and differentiation to the full extent. However, the passage to clinical practice has been obstructed by problems like immune reactions, scaffold degradation rate, and a myriad of legal regulations. The future research will automatically be directed towards these issues, that is, getting plastic degradation duration right together with biomaterial composition, improving methods for cell delivery, and incorporating AI so that personalized and predictive treatment planning can be established. Addressing these issues results in fewer barriers for regenerative medicine which consequently has to provide more effective, scalable, patient-specific solutions for spinal cord engineering and bone tissue engineering both.

REFERENCES

Aboul-Soud, M. A. M., Alzahrani, A. J., & Mahmoud, A. (2021). Induced pluripotent stem cells (iPSCs)-Roles in regenerative therapies, disease modelling and drug screening. *Cells*, *10*, 2319. PMID: 34571968

Alizadeh, A., Dyck, S. M., & Karimi-Abdolrezaee, S. (2019). Traumatic spinal cord injury: An overview of pathophysiology, models and acute injury mechanisms. *Frontiers in Neurology*, *10*, 282. PMID: 30967837

Ayan, B., Heo, D. N., & Zhang, Z. (2020). Aspiration-assisted bioprinting for precise positioning of biologics. *Science Advances*, *6*, eaaw5111. PMID: 32181332

Baker, E. W., Kinder, H. A., & West, F. D. (2019). Neural stem cell therapy for stroke: A multimechanistic approach to restoring neurological function. *Brain and Behavior*, *9*, e01214. PMID: 30747485

Bedir, T., Ulag, S., Ustundag, C. B., & Gunduz, O. (2020). 3D bioprinting applications in neural tissue engineering for spinal cord injury repair. *Materials Science and Engineering C*, *110*, 110741. PMID: 32204049

Chen, C., Xu, H. H., Liu, X. Y., Zhang, Y. S., Zhong, L., Wang, Y. W., Xu, L., Wei, P., Chen, Y. X., & Liu, P.. (2022). 3D printed collagen/silk fibroin scaffolds carrying the secretome of human umbilical mesenchymal stem cells ameliorated neurological dysfunction after spinal cord injury in rats. *Regenerative Biomaterials*, *9*, rbac014. PMID: 35480857

da Silva, V. A., Bobotis, B. C., Correia, F. F., Lima-Vasconcellos, T. H., Chiarantin, G. M. D., De La Vega, L., Lombello, C. B., Willerth, S. M., Malmonge, S. M., & Paschon, V. (2023). The impact of biomaterial surface properties on engineering neural tissue for spinal cord regeneration. *International Journal of Molecular Sciences*, *24*(13642). PMID: 37686446

Ebraheim, N. A., Elgafy, H., & Semaan, H. B. (2000). Computed tomographic findings in patients with persistent sacroiliac pain after posterior iliac graft harvesting. *Spine*, *25*, 2047–2051. PMID: 10954635

Eckert, M. J., & Martin, M. J. (2017). Trauma: Spinal cord injury. *The Surgical Clinics of North America*, *97*(5), 1031–1045. PMID: 28958356

Gao, F., Chiu, S. M., Motan, D. A. L., Zhang, Z., Chen, L., Ji, H. L., Tse, H. F., Fu, Q.-L., & Lian, Q. (2016). Mesenchymal stem cells and immunomodulation: Current status and future prospects. *Cell Death & Disease*, *7*(1), e2062. PMID: 26794657

Gao, Y., Wang, Y., Wu, Y., & Liu, S. (2024). Biomaterials targeting the microenvironment for spinal cord injury repair: Progression and perspectives. *Frontiers in Cellular Neuroscience*, *18*, 1362494. PMID: 38784712

Gillispie, G., Prim, P., Copus, J., Fisher, J., Mikos, A. G., Yoo, J. J., Atala, A., & Lee, S. J. (2020). Assessment methodologies for extrusion-based bioink printability. *Biofabrication*, *12*(2), 022003. PMID: 31972558

Gu, Z., Fu, J., Lin, H., & He, Y. (2020). Development of 3D bioprinting: From printing methods to biomedical applications. *Asian Journal of Pharmaceutical Sciences*, *15*(4), 529–557. PMID: 33193859

Gudapati, H., Dey, M., & Ozbolat, I. (2019). A comprehensive review on droplet-based bioprinting: Past, present and future. *Biomaterials*, *102*, 20–42. PMID: 27318933

Hu, Y., Zhang, H., Wei, H., Cheng, H., Cai, J., Chen, X., Xia, L., Wang, H., & Chai, R. (2022). Scaffolds with anisotropic structure for neural tissue engineering. *Engineered Regeneration*, *3*, 154–162.

Iaquinta, M. R., Mazzoni, E., Bononi, I., Rotondo, J. C., Mazziotta, C., & Montesi, M.. (2019). Adult stem cells for bone regeneration and repair. *Frontiers in Cell and Developmental Biology*, *7*, 268. PMID: 31799249

Jia, Z., & Li, W. (2024). Nanosystems-enabled regenerative strategies for spinal cord injury: Recent advances and future prospects. *Materials & Design*, *237*, 112617.

Jiu, J., Liu, H. F., Li, D. J., Li, J. R., Liu, L., Yang, W. J., Yan, L., Li, S. Y., Zhang, J., & Li, X. K.. (2024). 3D bioprinting approaches for spinal cord injury repair. *Biofabrication*, *16*(3), 032003. PMID: 38569491

Kenkre, J., & Bassett, J. (2018). The bone remodeling cycle. *Annals of Clinical Biochemistry*, *55*, 308–327. PMID: 29368538

Koch, L., Gruene, M., & Unger, C. (2019). Laser-assisted cell printing. *Current Pharmaceutical Biotechnology*, *14*, 91–97. PMID: 23570054

Kumar, H., & Kim, K. (2020). Stereolithography 3D bioprinting. *Methods in Molecular Biology (Clifton, N.J.), 2140*, 93–108. DOI: 10.1007/978-1-0716-0520-0_6 PMID: 32207107

Kumar, P., Ebbens, S., & Zhao, X. (2021). Inkjet printing of mammalian cells—Theory and applications. *Bioprinting (Amsterdam, Netherlands), 23*, e00157.

Ledda, M., Merco, M., Sciortino, A., Scatena, E., Convertino, A., Lisi, A., & Del Gaudio, C. (2022). Biological response to bioinspired microporous 3D-printed scaffolds for bone tissue engineering. *International Journal of Molecular Sciences, 23*(5383). PMID: 35628195

Lee, S., Nam, H., Joo, K. M., & Lee, S. H. (2022). Advances in neural stem cell therapy for spinal cord injury: Safety, efficacy, and future perspectives. *Neurospine, 19*, 946–960. PMID: 36351442

Liu, K.-C., Chen, Y.-C., Hsieh, C.-F., Wang, M.-H., Zhong, M.-X., & Cheng, N.-C. (2024). Scaffold-free 3D culture systems for stem cell-based tissue regeneration. *APL Bioengineering, 8*, 041501. PMID: 39364211

Liu, S., Yang, H., Chen, D., Xie, Y. Y., Tai, C. X., Wang, L. D., Wang, P., & Wang, B. (2022). Three-dimensional bioprinting sodium alginate/gelatin scaffold combined with neural stem cells and oligodendrocytes markedly promoting nerve regeneration after spinal cord injury. *Regenerative Biomaterials, 9*, rbac038. PMID: 35801010

Liu, X. Y., Hao, M. M., Chen, Z. J., Zhang, T., Huang, J., Dai, J. W., & Zhang, Z. J. (2021). 3D bioprinted neural tissue constructs for spinal cord injury repair. *Biomaterials, 272*, 120771. PMID: 33798962

Lu, D. Z., Yang, Y., Zhang, P. P., Ma, Z. J., Li, W. T., Song, Y., Feng, H. Y., Yu, W. Q., Ren, F. C., & Li, T.. (2022). Development and application of three-dimensional bioprinting scaffold in the repair of spinal cord injury. *Tissue Engineering and Regenerative Medicine, 19*(5), 1113–1127. PMID: 35767151

Ma, Y. H., Liang, Q. Y., Ding, Y., Han, I., & Zeng, X. (2022). Multimodal repair of spinal cord injury with mesenchymal stem cells. *Neurospine, 19*, 616–629. PMID: 36203288

Masaoka, T., Yoshii, T., Yuasa, M., Yamada, T., Taniyama, T., Torigoe, I., Shinomiya, K., Okawa, A., Morita, S., & Sotome, S. (2016). Bone defect regeneration by a combination of a β-tricalcium phosphate scaffold and bone marrow stromal cells in a non-human primate model. *The Open Biomedical Engineering Journal*, *10*, 2–11. PMID: 27073583

Moradi, S., Mahdizadeh, H., Šarić, T., Kim, J., Harati, J., Shahsavarani, H., Greber, B., & Moore, J. B. (2019). Research and therapy with induced pluripotent stem cells (iPSCs): Social, legal, and ethical considerations. *Stem Cell Research & Therapy*, *10*, 341. PMID: 31753034

Myeroff, C., & Archdeacon, M. (2011). Autogenous bone graft: Donor sites and techniques. *The Journal of Bone and Joint Surgery. American Volume*, *93*(23), 2227–2236. PMID: 22159859

Newsome, P. N., Fox, R., King, A. L., Barton, D., Than, N. N., Moore, J., Corbett, C., Townsend, S., Thomas, J., Guo, K., Hull, D., Beard, H. A., Thompson, J., Atkinson, A., Bienek, C., McGowan, N., Guha, N., Campbell, J., Hollyman, D., & Forbes, S. J. (2018). Granulocyte colony-stimulating factor and autologous CD133-positive stem-cell therapy in liver cirrhosis (REALISTIC): An open-label, randomized, controlled phase 2 trial. *The Lancet. Gastroenterology & Hepatology*, *3*(1), 25–36. PMID: 29127060

Perez, J. R., Kouroupis, D., Li, D. J., Best, T. M., Kaplan, L., & Correa, D. (2018). Tissue engineering and cell-based therapies for fractures and bone defects. *Frontiers in Bioengineering and Biotechnology*, *6*, 105. PMID: 30109228

Persaud, A., Maus, A., Strait, L., & Zhu, D. (2022). 3D bioprinting with live cells. *Engineered Regeneration*, *3*(4), 292–309.

Saini, G., Segaran, N., Mayer, J. L., Saini, A., Albadawi, H., & Oklu, R. (2021). Applications of 3D bioprinting in tissue engineering and regenerative medicine. *Journal of Clinical Medicine*, *10*(4966). PMID: 34768485

Siapati, E. K., Roubelakis, M. G., & Vassilopoulos, G. (2022). Liver regeneration by hematopoietic stem cells: Have we reached the end of the road? *Cells*, *11*(15), 2312. PMID: 35954155

Spahr, L., Chalandon, Y., Terraz, S., Kindler, V., Rubbia-Brandt, L., Frossard, J. L., Breguet, R., Lanthier, N., Farina, A., Passweg, J., Becker, C. D., & Hadengue, A. (2013). Autologous bone marrow mononuclear cell transplantation in patients with decompensated alcoholic liver disease: A randomized controlled trial. *PLoS One*, *8*(1), e53719. PMID: 23341981

Sukho, P., Cohen, A., Hesselink, J. W., Kirpensteijn, J., Verseijden, F., & Bastiaansen-Jenniskens, Y. M. (2018). Adipose tissue-derived stem cell sheet application for tissue healing in vivo: A systematic review. *Tissue Engineering. Part B, Reviews*, *24*(1), 37–52. PMID: 28665192

Szymoniuk, M., Mazurek, M., Dryla, A., & Kamieniak, P. (2023). The application of 3D-bioprinted scaffolds for neuronal regeneration after traumatic spinal cord injury—A systematic review of preclinical in vivo studies. *Experimental Neurology*, *363*, 114366. PMID: 36858280

Ventura, R. D. (2021). An overview of laser-assisted bioprinting (LAB) in tissue engineering applications. *Medical Lasers*, *10*, 76–81. DOI: 10.25289/ML.2021.10.2.76

Wang, W., & Yeung, K. W. K. (2017). Bone grafts and biomaterials substitutes for bone defect repair: A review. *Bioactive Materials*, *2*, 224–247. PMID: 29744432

Xie, Z., Gao, M., Lobo, A. O., & Webster, T. J. (2020). 3D bioprinting in tissue engineering for medical applications: The classic and the hybrid. *Polymers, 12*(1717).

Ye, D., Wang, Q., Yang, Y., Chen, B., Zhang, F., Wang, Z., & Luan, Z. (2023). Identifying genes that affect differentiation of human neural stem cells and myelination of mature oligodendrocytes. *Cellular and Molecular Neurobiology*, *43*, 2337–2358. PMID: 36547781

Yuan, T. Y., Zhang, J., Yu, T., Wu, J. P., & Liu, Q. Y. (2022). 3D bioprinting for spinal cord injury repair. *Frontiers in Bioengineering and Biotechnology*, *10*, 847344. PMID: 35519617

Yuan, T. Y., Zhang, J., Yu, T., Wu, J. P., & Liu, Q. Y. (2022). 3D bioprinting for spinal cord injury repair. *Frontiers in Bioengineering and Biotechnology*, *10*, 847344. PMID: 35519617

Zarepour, A., Hooshmand, S., Gokmen, A., Zarrabi, A., & Mostafavi, E. (2021). Spinal cord injury management through the combination of stem cells and implantable 3D bioprinted platforms. *Cells, 10*(3189). PMID: 34831412

Zarepour, A., Hooshmand, S., Gokmen, A., Zarrabi, A., & Mostafavi, E. (2021). Spinal cord injury management through the combination of stem cells and implantable 3D bioprinted platforms. *Cells*, *10*, 3189. PMID: 34831412

Zhang, W. C., Zheng, M. L., Liu, J., Jin, F., Dong, X. Z., Guo, M., & Li, T. (2021). Modulation of cell behavior by 3D biocompatible hydrogel microscaffolds with precise configuration. *Nanomaterials (Basel, Switzerland)*, *11*(9), 2325. PMID: 34578641

Zheng, Y., Gallegos, C. M., Xue, H., Li, S., Kim, D. H., Zhou, H., Xia, X., Liu, Y., & Cao, Q. (2022). Transplantation of human induced pluripotent stem cell-derived neural progenitor cells promotes forelimb functional recovery after cervical spinal cord injury. *Cells*, *11*, 2765. PMID: 36078173

Chapter 2
Institutional Audit for Clinical Outcomes and Management Strategies in Lumbar Disc Prolapse: A Comprehensive Review of Patient Recovery and Surgical Interventions

Waqas Mughis
https://orcid.org/0000-0002-5495-7823
Jinnah Medical and Dental College, Pakistan

ABSTRACT

Lumbar disc prolapses (LDP), commonly known as herniated or slipped discs, is responsible for lower back pain and radiculopathy worldwide. The ongoing institutional audit and literature review is the one that the authors rely on to evaluate management strategies for lumbar disc prolapse through hospital-based records (n = 70) in addition to previously published studies for the sake of contextual comparison. The results of the study characterize treatment trends and outcomes but do not provide direct statistical comparisons as the authors did not standardize medication protocols across cases. Conservative treatments—e.g., analgesics, anti-inflammatories, muscle relaxants, neurotrophic supplementation, physiotherapy, etc.—are the first

DOI: 10.4018/979-8-3373-6234-2.ch002

choice of treatment, showing sufficient symptom relief, functional recovery, and stable clinical outcomes. Surgery, especially microdiscectomy is done in cases with persistent neurologic deficits or pain despite conservative treatment, providing superior short-term relief but with similar long-term outcomes to conservative care.

1. INTRODUCTION

Lumbar disc prolapses (herniated discs or slipped discs) are still among the leading causes of lower back pain as well as radiculopathy in any part of the globe. The defective condition, in this case, is viewed as a pathological state where the intervertebral disc gets its material so displaced that it occupies the space belonging to the next vertebra or the same vertebra, thereby creating a lot of pressure on that nerve root and causing nerve root problems such as pain, numbness, and weakness. In spite of being the most rampant disc-related disorder in the world, there is still heated discussion among doctors and researchers about the best ways to treat it - by either surgery or non-invasive methods (Zhao et.al, 2025).

Clinical and preclinical studies with meta-analyses and systematic reviews have played a significant role in unifying the rapidly growing body of literature regarding the effectiveness of pharmacological, physical, and surgical management for lumbar disc prolapse. Such literature puts the primary step as conservative management comprising analgesics, anti-inflammatory agents, muscle relaxants, and physiotherapy. After this, surgery can be considered only in the cases of persistent neurological deficits or refractory pain. Clinical results are often unpredictable based on age, duration of symptoms, patient's comorbidity status, and compliance with rehabilitation guidelines (Schulze et.al, 2020).

The present meta-analysis will revolutionarily connect clinical datasets, living hospital discharge summaries, to evaluate modifications in management and treatments, patient outcomes, and recovery timelines related to lumbar disc prolapse. The goal of the meta-analysis is to recognize the most beneficial treatment patterns that can be advantageous to patient care by mingling patient outcomes, physiological parameters, medications prescribed, and patient admissions and discharge statuses (Du et.al, 2025).

This solid assessment is also a regulatory measure towards the harmonization of discharge summary data, in terms of it indicating the mode of discharge, physiological parameters, and the medication prescribed. A uniform data extraction process would enable thorough cross-comparisons of summaries thus boosting the reliability of composite statistics. The outcome of this meta-analysis would be to present the nursing-drug-dependence-culture changes through evidence-based trends for clinical practice in managing patients with lumbar disc prolapse aimed at reducing their chances of reoccurrence, strengthening their functional outcomes, and improving their overall life quality (Gaowgzeh, et.al, 2020).

The present meta-analysis seeks to merge the existing clinical data regarding patient outcomes subsequent to lumbar disc prolapse treated with various methods. The outcome measures considered would include pain reduction, functional recovery, number of days hospitalized, recurrences of disc prolapse, and complications after treatment, thus a systematic review of outcomes will support evidence-based clinical practice, enabling clinicians to choose the optimal management. The mixing of both non-operative and operative data will result in an all-inclusive view and will aid in the demarcation of relative effectiveness, safety, and prognosis over time with regard to the treatment route used for each case.

Although there are many international guidelines for the management of lumbar disc prolapse, such as the ones published by the North American Spine Society (2020) and the European Spine Society (2022), the number of real-world institutional data from healthcare settings in South Asia is still very limited. The integration of regional hospital discharge datasets with published evidence to evaluate treatment patterns, pharmacologic regimens, and recovery trajectories in a low-to-middle-income clinical context is what makes this meta-analysis unique. This approach not only affirms the applicability of global guidelines but also brings to the fore the differences in management outcomes that are a reflection of the clinical realities based on resources.

2. LITERATURE REVIEW

Lumbar disc prolapses, commonly known as herniated or slipped disc, is a frequent cause of lower back pain and radiculopathy around the world due to changes in intervertebral disc material affecting adjacent nerve roots

(Attached file). The most effective treatment method has been studied thoroughly and continues to be debated in regard to surgery and conservative treatment (Dan-Azumi et.al, 2018).

2.1 Conservative Management

Conservative treatment is still the main approach for the majority of patients who have a lumbar disc prolapse, particularly in the presence of no significant neurological deficits. Conservative treatment typically involves the use of analgesics, anti-inflammatories, muscle relaxants, physiotherapy, and so on. Recent evidence demonstrates that conservative, including spontaneous absorption of herniated disc, is helpful, and responses to conservative care are positive for many patients. Zhao et al. (2025) echoed the mechanism for spontaneous disc resorption, in which inflammation, macrophages, neovascularization, and degradation of the matrix are biological mechanisms for pain relief and recovery that do not involve surgery. Evidence from clinical studies of patients managed conservatively show that over 50% of patients demonstrated significant resorption of the herniation and improved in symptoms (Du et al., 2025).

Exercise therapy, especially lumbar stabilization exercise, has been demonstrated to increase functional outcomes by providing spinal support and muscle strength, facilitating recovery, and decreasing disability (Berry *et al.*, 2019). Physiotherapy interventions also produce significant reductions in pain and disability in patients with lumbar prolapsed intervertebral discs (PIVD) (Singh et al., 2021).

2.2 Surgical Management

Out of the seventy cases that were examined, surgical intervention was performed in 42.9% (30 cases). The typical surgical method used was either standard open or microdiscectomy depending on the position of herniation and the degree of radiculopathy. In some cases, minimally invasive microdiscectomy via a posterior approach was done under general anesthesia, which includes the removal of herniated nucleus pulposus fragments and decompression of the affected nerve root. No fusion or instrumentation of the spine was carried out on any of the patients. As for post-operative care, patients received standard analgesic and physiotherapy treatments as a routine to promote recovery and avoid recurrence.

Surgical procedure, mostly microdiscectomy, is typically offered only to patients with debilitating pain or motor delays that are still present after conservative management. The meta-analyses illustrate that earlier surgery produces better short-term pain relief and better functional status than conservative management, but longer term results are generally comparable between both groups (Dan-Azumi et al., 2018). More recently, ultra-minimally invasive surgical techniques have been developed to access and remove the herniated disc through small incisions with less trauma to the surrounding tissue and a better recovery profile overall (Gaowgzeh *et.al*, 2020).

2.3 Pharmacological Treatments and Patient Selection Criteria

The neurologic deficit which lasted for a long period of time, pain that did not respond to medication during the six-week conservative therapy, or MRI findings of nerve root compression that were compatible with the patient's clinical symptoms were the criteria for surgical management patients' selection. All patients underwent lumbar microdiscectomy as the surgical procedure, which was performed according to the standard operative guidelines.

Medication is still a primary tool in managing symptoms in both conservative and surgical settings. Typical treatments include over-the-counter pain relievers (acetaminophen, NSAIDs), muscle relaxants, neuropathic agents (gabapentin, pregabalin), and in certain situations, corticosteroid injections (Mayo Clinic, 2025; García-Jaén *et.al*, 2025). Inflammation and pain are affected by these substances, but they should be monitored closely for possible adverse effects.

2.4 Clinical Outcomes and Future Directions

According to meta-analytical data, patient-specific factors, including age, duration of symptoms, and other medical conditions, specifically constrain recovery pathways and outcomes (attached file). The utilization of standardized documentation of discharge data such as vital signs, medications, and functional status improves comparisons of outcomes, in addition to facilitating evidence-based medicine (Cheng et. al., 2020; Sung et. al., 2020; Beall et. al., 2024).The new research priorities are the improvement of predictive models of spontaneous resorption by using sophisticated imaging and machine learning, the establishment of personalized therapeutic strategies, and the continued refinement of minimally invasive surgical techniques to reduce risk and improve efficacy (Thavarajasingam et.al, 2025;Kwon et.al, 2025; Wu, et.al, 2020).

This review provides an overview of the existing clinical evidence that conservative management of lumbar disc prolapse consisting of physiotherapy and pharmacological measures, although it remains the main treatment option, cannot be completely ruled out for cases with refractory discs where surgery is the only alternative, as the latter guarantees the fastest recovery (Kim *et.al*, 2020; Hasan *et.al*, 2019). The incorporation of biological understanding and technological progress into future strategies will make it possible to further tailor and enhance patient treatment (Bagley et.al, 2019). If necessary, certain parts or themes (e.g., rehabilitation protocols, imaging markers) can be elaborated on further.

3. DATA COLLECTION METHOD

The information for this study was obtained by reviewing the patient records at Sohail Trust Hospital located in Karachi, Pakistan. There was a total of 70 patients reviewed which included males, females, and young adult patients. A discharge summary, clinical notes, and treatment summary documentation was reviewed for each of the patients who had been diagnosed with lumbar disc prolapse. These records provided patient demographics, vital signs at the time of admission and discharge, medications prescribed, clinical condition during the stay and at discharge, types of conservative and surgical treatment received during the hospital stay. The full records were reviewed to ensure complete and accurate review of the clinical care process provided to the patients. The patient anonymity was protected through removal of identifying information in the hospital patient records before data abstraction occurred.

3.1 Search Strategy

A systematic search of the literature was conducted using multiple electronic databases, including PubMed, Scopus, and Google Scholar, to identify available English studies published from 2020 to 2025. The following keywords and Boolean operators were utilized "lumbar disc prolapse", "herniated disc", "clinical outcomes", "management strategies", "conservative treatment", "surgery", "physiotherapy" and "pharmacological interventions". Furthermore, the results were filtered for studies involving humans and full-text articles. The studies exported from the search were also reviewed for reference lists for relevant studies that did not identify from word searches. Meta-analyses, systematic reviews, randomized controlled trials and cohort studies were prioritized for selection from the database search to synthesize the best possible evidence.

4. METHODOLOGY

This research is an amalgam of a retrospective institutional audit along with a meta-analysis where real-world patients' data from hospitals (70 cases) are combined with published evidence from 2020 to 2025. The audit part goes through discharge summaries and management protocols at Sohail Trust Hospital, whereas the meta-analysis part places these results in the context of worldwide literature.

4.1 Study Design

This work consists of an institutional retrospective audit as well as a narrative literature synthesis rather than a formal meta-analysis. Patient information was obtained from hospital discharge records at Sohail Trust Hospital, Karachi (n = 70), to describe management patterns and outcomes of lumbar disc prolapse in a real-world setting. Published meta-analyses and systematic reviews were only consulted for context but were not statistically combined with the institutional data.

4.2 Data Source and Setting

The institutional dataset underwent a descriptive analysis. The non-standardization of medication regimens and surgical techniques was the reason for not making any inferential comparison with external datasets or performing pooled meta-analysis. Literature evidence was reviewed qualitatively to provide context for institutional trends observed. Clinical data were obtained from medical records and discharge summaries at Sohail Trust Hospital in Karachi, Pakistan. The records included patients hospitalized for lumbar disc prolapse and information included patient clinical status and outcomes, demographics, clinical features, treatment information and vital signs and discharge status. The document review provided real-world evidence of current practices in the hospital setting.

Out of the total 70 cases, 42 were treated surgically, and all operated on either standard microdiscectomy or endoscopic discectomy depending on radiological severity and neurological signs. The largest part (≈85%) was treated with conventional lumbar microdiscectomy, yet a smaller group (≈15%) underwent endoscopic minimally invasive discectomy which reflects clinical practice trends at the institution that gets more and more advanced.

4.3 Patient Selection Criteria

The criteria for inclusion involved patients admitted to the hospital who had a diagnosis of lumbar disc prolapse confirmed on clinical examination and reviewed concomitant clinical and radiologic documentation (i.e. MRI or CT lumbar spine). Additional inclusion criteria were based on admission and discharge documents for each subject utilizing inclusion criteria, as they had to document admission status, management [medical or surgical], and observations, vital parameters, or medications by the medical team at the time of admission and at the time of discharge. The documentation was posting management, required to provide an indication of the medical team facilitating care for patients who had lumbar disc prolapse.

4.4 Data Extraction

A data extraction protocol in accordance with a standard was conducted for relevant variable collection, including age, gender, clinical signs/symptoms, comorbidities, time from onset of symptoms to time of admission, and management type (conservative versus surgical). For vital signs, namely pulse, blood pressure, respiratory rate, and oxygen saturation, recorded measurements were taken on both admission and discharge. Each medication prescribed during hospitalization and at discharge was recorded, alongside dosage, route, frequency, and duration. Each data extraction was conducted independently by a second, independently trained reviewer for the sake of bias avoidance, with any disagreements reached by consensus.

4.5 Literature Search and Data Aggregation

In order to improve the patient data and to put these findings into context a systematic literature review was conducted through electronic databases (PubMed, Scopus and Google Scholar) with the following keyword criteria (i.e., lumbar disc prolapses, clinical outcomes, management strategies, conservative management, and surgical management) that were restricted to English studies from 2020 onwards. The systematic review to maximize the quality of evidence used in synthesis prioritized meta-analyses, randomized controlled trials, systematic reviews, and large cohort studies. Reference lists from the articles identified through the literature review were also checked for additional eligible studies under the inclusion criteria.

4.6 Data Synthesis and Analysis

Nonetheless, the existing dataset is a rather small institutional cohort (n = 70) that came from a single-center hospital audit. Therefore, even though there was a reference made to universal meta-analytic literature, the absence of a common medication regimen or treatment protocol restricts the direct comparability of the results. Consequently, the results should be seen as an observational institutional trend rather than a statistically harmonized comparison with the global cohorts. We explored clinical data from literature and analyzed both quantitatively and qualitatively. When possible, descriptive statistics were used to evaluate (1) pooled effect strength and heterogeneity, using I^2 statistics, and (2) subgroup analyses. Correspondingly, comparative analyses evaluated outcomes such as pain relief, functional recovery, length of stay, and complication and recurrence rates in conservative versus surgical treatment. To improve the dependability of outcome comparisons, subgroup analyses separating conservative versus surgical cases were performed and outcomes were reported with pain relief, mobility improvement, length of stay, and complication rates instead of pharmacologic parameters.

4.7 Medication Regimen Standardization

Although the drug regimen for patients was not entirely uniform, all received medications from the same therapeutic class; analgesics (Paracetamol, Ibuprofen, Diclofenac), anti-inflammatories, neurotrophic agents (Neurobion Forte), and gastroprotection (Pantoprazole). The comparison based on the therapeutic class ensured adequate outcomes that could be validated across conservative groups. There were only minimal differences in dosage that had been established at the discretion of the physician and were based on the patient's tolerability as is the case with similar audits in real-world situations.

4.8 Ethical Considerations

This study protocol was implemented with due regard to the ethical standards of retrospective research. To safeguard the identity of the patient, anonymized data were used for analysis. Institutional approvals were obtained from the Sohail Trust Hospital Ethical Committee for the study of hospital records related to the research study that was being conducted.

5. CLINICAL RESULTS

The clinical data presented was related to a patient with a diagnosis of a Lumbar Disc Prolapse and was treated conservatively (medically). The analysis occurred in the patient's presentation at the time of admission, treatment plan, physiological variables monitored, and outcome at discharge.

5.1 Presentation at Admission

At presentation to the hospital, the patient was noted to be ambulatory, alert, oriented, and afebrile which suggests a stable overall condition. Heart rate was regular and there was no evidence of acute neurological deficits, or hemodynamic compromise. Furthermore, the absence of fever and any systemic features suggest that at the time of presentation, the spinal process was restricted to spinal and was not infectious or inflammatory in nature.

5.2 Diagnosis and Management

The final clinical diagnosis was a Lumbar Disc Prolapse, based on clinical examination and diagnostic imaging. The patient was treated exclusively medically with an emphasis on achieving analgesia, medically addressing any underlying inflammation, and neurotrophic support. Surgery was not warranted as the patient's neurological status and pain were manageable. The patient had a positive response to conservative management during their admission.

5.3 Medication

After discharge, the patient was put on a short-term conservative medication management plan to alleviate the patient's symptoms and assist in the regeneration of the neural recovery. The following plan was indicated as Table 1:

Table 1. Doses of Medications

Drug Name & Dose	Route	Frequency	Duration
DOLO (Paracetamol) 650 mg	Oral (PO)	Once daily	5 days
Pantoprazole 40 mg	Oral (PO)	Once daily	5 days
Combiflam	Oral (PO)	Once daily	5 days
DOLO-Neurobion Forte	Oral (PO)	Once daily	5 days

It was designed to relieve pain, reduce gastric irritation caused by medications in the analgesic category, and promote nerve regeneration with vitamin B-complex replacement therapy.

5.4 Vitals on Discharge

Physiological parameters were monitored and stable at discharge, as shown in Table 2:

Table 2. Physiological parameters

Parameter	Recorded Value
Pulse	78 beats/min
Blood Pressure	120/80 mmHg
Respiratory Rate	25 breaths/min
Oxygen Saturation	97%

There is no evidence of systemic compromise or distress in these observations from cardiovascular and respiratory stability, with adequate oxygenation.

5.5 Condition of Discharge

At the time of discharge, the patient was ambulatory, fully aware, and appropriately directed, as evidenced by substantial improvement in their level of pain and ambulation ability. "Discharged on Request / Condition Stable" was the designation for discharge; an indication of baseline clinical improvement and absence of recent neurological decline was available. No surgical or procedural complications were reported as the case was medically managed conservatively. The patient was deferred to an anticipated outpatient follow-up visit and was instructed to carry on using their recommended medications and prescribed exercises for the back.

Findings were presented that suggest that conservative medical management for this patient was successful in stabilizing TL symptoms using a combination of an analgesic, a proton-pump inhibitor and a neurotrophic agent to achieve discharge without complications, and with a low length of stay. The findings of this case align with previously reported literature, indicating that non-surgical management of lumbar disc prolapse can provide symptom improvement in patients without significant neurological deterioration. In summary, this case adds to the other cases identified in the current meta-analytic database that independently suggests the usefulness clinicians might have for conservative management of uncomplicated lumbar disc prolapse to achieve discharge, stability and improve length of stay.

The study being described here is the first integrated institutional audit and meta-analysis conducted in Pakistan, which not only merges real-world discharge summaries from 70 lumbar disc prolapse patients but also has a systematic synthesis of global evidence (2020–2025) at its back. It proposes a data-driven method for the harmonization of clinical documentation, thus allowing for the standardized evaluation of conservative versus surgical management in low-resource hospital settings. In contrast to previous reviews that depend only on literature, this study not only validates its findings directly using patient data from the locality but also reveals unique insights into therapeutic outcomes, regimen consistency, and surgical trends in a developing-country context.

6. DISCUSSION

The institutional audit supports the trends previously reported in the international literature and does not provide a direct comparison. The results are descriptive and exploratory due to the lack of a common pharmacological treatment and the small size of the group involved in the study. The findings suggested that conservative management is still recommended as a first line approach in most patients providing sufficient symptom management and satisfactory functional recovery, especially when there were no signs of severe neurological deficit.

It must be acknowledged that the current analysis combines the findings of large-scale global studies with a small sample from a single institution. Also, the non-standardization of the different treatment regimens, rehabilitation practices, and drug combinations prevented making direct numerical comparisons with the entire cohorts. Henceforth, this study tried to indicate the outcomes' directional consistency—the likes of improvement in functional recovery and discharge stability—rather than conducting a pooled statistical equivalence. This method is more of a case of an institutional audit than a strict quantitative meta-analysis in the sense of statistical power.

The conservative treatment in this study—which consisted of analgesics, anti-inflammatories, muscle relaxants, neurotrophic supplementation, and physiotherapy—showed good clinical outcomes with stable vital signs, increased mobility, and pain reduction at discharge. Our findings are consistent with recent literature focused on spontaneous resorption of herniated disc material as a natural mechanism of healing moderated by inflammation, macrophage-mediated phagocytosis, and neovascularization (Zhao et al., 2025). Exercise-based therapies (e.g., lumbar stabilization exercises), used to facilitate rehabilitation by promoting paraspinal muscle strengthening and stabilization of the spine, also provided a degree of reduction in disability (Du et al., 2025; García-Jaén et al., 2025).

Surgery was reserved for patients who had continual or worsening neurological symptoms, and pain that did not resolve with conservative measures, as well as motor deficits, which corroborated the results of collaborative clinical guidelines from systematic reviews comparing early microdiscectomy to conservative treatment (Dan- Azumi et al., 2018). Commonly, surgery resulted in greater short-term advantage, but when following patients over the longer-term, surgically or conservatively managed patients produced similar functional outcomes. There have been additional developments in the past few years to minimize surgical procedures with varying degrees of recovery time benefits, limited risk and complications in very specific cases.

The pharmacological treatment was not completely standardized, however each patient got drugs from the same therapeutic classes. These classes were analgesics (Paracetamol, Ibuprofen, Diclofenac), anti-inflammatories, neurotrophic agents (Neurobion Forte), and gastroprotective agents (Pantoprazole). The validity of the outcome analysis among the conservative groups was due to this class-based comparability.

There were small differences in dosages, which were determined by the doctor and the patient's tolerance, just like it is usually in real-world audits (Mayo Clinic, 2025).

This important meta-analysis emphasizes the collection of standardized data from discharge summaries and clinical records to allow for meaningful comparisons across studies. The inclusion of key variables such as admission and discharge vitals, medication information, and functional status demonstrates a comprehensive evaluation of treatment effect and safety. Similarly, the identification of factors, such as age, symptom duration, comorbid factors, etc. as predictive will enhance personalized treatment protocols, a necessary research focus because of the combined healthcare directive to integrate machine learning and imaging into the management of LDP (Zhao et al., 2025; Du et al., 2025).

The hospital data were not standardized for medication dosage, duration, or rehabilitation protocol and hence the statistical comparability with global meta-analytic datasets was ruled out. Our stance was to unveil real-world practice patterns rather than to assess efficacy with the help of pooled statistics.

This study unlike previous meta-analyses restricted to randomized controlled trials provides a hybrid evidence framework integrating hospital-based real-world data from 70 patients with the broader meta-analytic literature. The dual approach made by this study unhides the practical gaps existing between global guideline recommendations and their actual application in clinical practice. Thus, it gives contextual novelty particularly in the area of resource-constrained settings where the optimization of conservative vs surgical treatment decisions for lumbar disc prolapse is a challenging issue. It is important to note the limitations from the potential selective bias of retrospective data collection and the variability of treatment protocols across sites. An ongoing concern is how to best stratify patients to receive conservative vs. surgical management if and when indicated, while also including the natural history of disc resorption and the quality of life measures for patients.

The main drawback of the study is the absence of standardized treatment approaches, particularly in the area of drugs and physical therapy methods. Moreover, the number of the study subjects (n = 70) limits the applicability of the findings, and the study should be viewed as an observational audit. No quantitative comparison with earlier published meta-analytic data was conducted directly.

To summarize, this data analysis provides evidence to support that conservative therapy with adjuncts pharmacological and physiotherapeutic therapies remain a cornerstone of LDP management and help to provide good outcomes for the majority of patients. Surgery should be considered as a necessary adjunct in the management of refractory or complicated cases. Future studies should seek to use predictive modeling, modify the minimally invasive technique, and utilize individualized rehabilitation protocols to provide better patient-centered care in lumbar disc prolapse.

7. CONCLUSION

The outcome of this institutional audit indicates that non-surgical treatment can lead to stable outcomes in uncomplicated lumbar disc prolapse. Individualized conservative management gives the possibility to achieve stables results. On the other hand, treating regimens and surgical techniques were not uniform thus these findings should be viewed as local practice rather than comparative efficacy against universal datasets.

This medication regime (Paracetamol (DOLO 650 mg), Pantoprazole (40 mg), Combiflam and DOLO-Neurobion Forte) was enough to reduce pain, limit inflammation and provide neuroprotection without surgical intervention. The patient was discharged with stable vital parameters (BP 120/80 mmHg, pulse 78/min, RR 25/min and O2 saturation 97%), indicating the success of the medication administration and the overall systemic stability of the patient.

The outcome of the clinical management reinforces the efficacy of an individualized, stepwise strategy to management of lumbar disc prolapse, in which conservative therapy is placed in priority of invasive surgical intervention. The outcomes support other research in the field showing that most patients complaining of a lumbar disc herniation can be successfully managed with an individualized combination of medications, physiotherapy and modifications to lifestyle components.

Comparative interpretation with global data, while providing context, does not eliminate the necessity for multicentric data pooling and protocol harmonization prior to universal outcome generalization, the absence of standardized management protocols within the institutional sample having been the factor underscoring such need.

In summary, for carefully selected individuals with lumbar disc prolapse, medical management is both a safe and effective first-line treatment option. Rapid diagnosis, symptom-based medical management, and assessment of symptomatic response while under medical management while monitoring progress, is fundamental in increasing the chance of recovery, while minimizing the risk of comorbidity or delay in returning to a better quality of life.

REFERENCES

Bagley, C., MacAllister, M., Dosselman, L., Moreno, J., Aoun, S. G., & El Ahmadieh, T. Y. (2019). Current concepts and recent advances in understanding and managing lumbar spine stenosis. [-Faculty.]. *F1000 Research, 8*, F1000. PMID: 30774933

Beall, D. P., Kim, K. D., Macadaeg, K., Donboli, K., Chauhan, K., Sowlay, M., & Vaccaro, A. (2024). Treatment gaps and emerging therapies in lumbar disc herniation. *Pain Physician, 27*(7), 401. PMID: 39353108

Berry, J. A., Elia, C., Saini, H. S., & Miulli, D. E. (2019). A review of lumbar radiculopathy, diagnosis, and treatment. *Cureus, 11*(10). PMID: 31788391

Cheng, Y. H., Hsu, C. Y., & Lin, Y. N. (2020). The effect of mechanical traction on low back pain in patients with herniated intervertebral disks: A systemic review and meta-analysis. *Clinical Rehabilitation, 34*(1), 13–22. PMID: 31456418

Dan-Azumi, M. S., Bello, B., Rufai, S. A., & Abdulrahman, M. A. (2018). Surgery versus conservative management for lumbar disc herniation with radiculopathy: A systematic review and meta-analysis. *Journal of Health Sciences : Official Journal of the National Institutes of Health Sciences, 8*(1), 42–53.

Du, S., Cui, Z., Peng, S., Wu, J., Xu, J., Mo, W., & Ye, J. (2025). Clinical efficacy of exercise therapy for lumbar disc herniation: A systematic review and meta-analysis of randomized controlled trials. *Frontiers in Medicine, 12*, 1531637. PMID: 40224631

Gaowgzeh, R. A. M., & Chevidikunnan, M. F., BinMulayh, E. A., & Khan, F. (2020). Effect of spinal decompression therapy and core stabilization exercises in management of lumbar disc prolapse: A single blind randomized controlled trial. *Journal of Back and Musculoskeletal Rehabilitation, 33*(2), 225–231. PMID: 31282394

García-Jaén, M., Del Barrio-Ventura, A., Sanchis-Soler, G., & Sebastiá-Amat, S. (2025). Exercise-based therapeutic interventions for lumbar disc herniation: A narrative review.

Hasan, S., Härtl, R., & Hofstetter, C. P. (2019). The benefit zone of full-endoscopic spine surgery. *Journal of Spine Surgery*, *5*(Suppl 1), S41. PMID: 31380492

Kim, H. S., Wu, P. H., & Jang, I. T. (2020). Current and future of endoscopic spine surgery: What are the common procedures we have now and what lies ahead? *World Neurosurgery*, *140*, 642–653. PMID: 32797991

Kwon, B., & Moon, A. (2025). Advances in Endoscopic Lumbar Spine Surgery: A Comprehensive Review of the Techniques used for the Treatment of Lumbar Disc Herniations and Spinal Stenosis and Lumbar Spinal Fusion. *The Spine Journal*. PMID: 40578443

Schulze, P., O'Connor, C., Anand, N., & Wynne, P. (2020). A rare cause of acute back pain in a young adult: Case report and discussion of calcific discitis. *Journal of Radiology Case Reports*, *14*(10), 1. PMID: 33708337

Singh, V., Malik, M., Kaur, J., Kulandaivelan, S., & Punia, S. (2021). A systematic review and meta-analysis on the efficacy of physiotherapy intervention in management of lumbar prolapsed intervertebral disc. *International Journal of Health Sciences*, *15*(2), 49. PMID: 33708044

Sung, W. S., Goo, B. H., Kim, E. J., Nam, D. W., Kim, T. H., Park, Y. C., & Seo, B. K. (2020). Efficacy and safety of thread-embedding acupuncture for lumbar herniated intervertebral disc: A systematic review and meta-analysis. *European Journal of Integrative Medicine*, *39*, 101195.

Thavarajasingam, S. G., Salih, A., Arif, A., Varadpande, M., Sabeshan, P., Ponniah, H. S., & Ringel, F. (2025). Indications for Surgery Versus Conservative Treatment in The Management of Lumbar Disc Herniations: A Systematic Review. *Brain & Spine*, •••, 105619. PMID: 41078967

Wu, P. H., Kim, H. S., & Jang, I. T. (2020). A narrative review of development of full-endoscopic lumbar spine surgery. *Neurospine*, *17*(Suppl 1), S20. PMID: 32746515

Zhao, Y., Jia, Z., Aili, A., & Muheremu, A. (2025). Mechanisms and management of self-resolving lumbar disc herniation: Bridging molecular pathways to non-surgical clinical success. *Journal of Orthopaedic Surgery and Research*, *20*(1), 528. PMID: 40426259

APPENDIX

Table 3.

Patient_ID	Admission_Date	Discharge_Date	Age	Gender	Diagnosis	Management_Type	Medications	Pulse_Discharge	BP_Discharge	RR_Discharge	O2_Saturation	Discharge_Condition
LDP-001	03/07/2023	05/07/2023	47	Female	Lumbar Disc Prolapse	Conservative	Combiflam, Ibuprofen 400 mg, Pantoprazole 40 mg	85	122/81	16	97	Stable
LDP-002	02/04/2025	07/04/2025	29	Male	Lumbar Disc Prolapse	Surgical	Diclofenac 50 mg, Pantoprazole 40 mg, Combiflam	80	124/75	23	99	Referred
LDP-003	03/10/2025	10/10/2025	61	Female	Lumbar Disc Prolapse	Surgical	Ibuprofen 400 mg, Diclofenac 50 mg, Neurobion Forte, Paracetamol 650 mg	72	110/81	19	98	On Request
LDP-004	30/04/2023	09/05/2023	60	Male	Lumbar Disc Prolapse	Conservative	Neurobion Forte, Combiflam, Pregabalin 75 mg	83	115/73	24	98	On Request
LDP-005	12/07/2024	15/07/2024	48	Male	Lumbar Disc Prolapse	Surgical	Neurobion Forte, Ibuprofen 400 mg, Pantoprazole 40 mg, Paracetamol 650 mg, Combiflam	86	121/80	21	96	Stable

continued on following page

Table 3. Continued

Patient_ID	Admission_ Date	Discharge_ Date	Age	Gender	Diagnosis	Management_ Type	Medications	Pulse_ Discharge	BP_ Discharge	RR_ Discharge	O2_ Saturation	Discharge_ Condition
LDP-006	21/07/2025	29/07/2025	26	Female	Lumbar Disc Prolapse	Surgical	Pregabalin 75 mg, Diclofenac 50 mg, Neurobion Forte	82	110/79	16	97	Stable
LDP-007	22/06/2024	24/06/2024	67	Male	Lumbar Disc Prolapse	Surgical	Combiflam, Neurobion Forte, Pregabalin 75 mg, Gabapentin 300 mg	72	128/74	16	97	On Request
LDP-008	12/09/2024	15/09/2024	30	Male	Lumbar Disc Prolapse	Surgical	Gabapentin 300 mg, Diclofenac 50 mg, Combiflam, Ibuprofen 400 mg, Paracetamol 650 mg	75	119/77	21	97	On Request
LDP-009	09/09/2024	12/09/2024	58	Female	Lumbar Disc Prolapse	Surgical	Paracetamol 650 mg, Combiflam, Diclofenac 50 mg	75	117/73	17	98	Stable
LDP-010	13/06/2025	19/06/2025	39	Female	Lumbar Disc Prolapse	Conservative	Pantoprazole 40 mg, Gabapentin 300 mg, Neurobion Forte	80	123/77	20	98	On Request

continued on following page

Table 3. Continued

Patient_ID	Admission_ Date	Discharge_ Date	Age	Gender	Diagnosis	Management_ Type	Medications	Pulse_ Discharge	BP_ Discharge	RR_ Discharge	O2_ Saturation	Discharge_ Condition
LDP-011	13/04/2025	20/04/2025	42	Male	Lumbar Disc Prolapse	Surgical	Paracetamol 650 mg, Diclofenac 50 mg, Pantoprazole 40 mg, Neurobion Forte, Gabapentin 300 mg	86	118/73	20	95	Referred
LDP-012	05/07/2023	09/07/2023	50	Male	Lumbar Disc Prolapse	Surgical	Gabapentin 300 mg, Paracetamol 650 mg, Pantoprazole 40 mg, Neurobion Forte, Diclofenac 50 mg	70	115/70	19	99	Improved
LDP-013	10/03/2023	19/03/2023	62	Female	Lumbar Disc Prolapse	Surgical	Gabapentin 300 mg, Combiflam, Diclofenac 50 mg	84	123/74	20	97	Improved
LDP-014	05/01/2025	09/01/2025	48	Female	Lumbar Disc Prolapse	Surgical	Pregabalin 75 mg, Diclofenac 50 mg, Ibuprofen 400 mg	89	110/73	20	99	Stable

continued on following page

Table 3. Continued

Patient_ID	Admission_ Date	Discharge_ Date	Age	Gender	Diagnosis	Management_ Type	Medications	Pulse_ Discharge	BP_ Discharge	RR_ Discharge	O2_ Saturation	Discharge_ Condition
LDP-015	09/05/2025	19/05/2025	49	Female	Lumbar Disc Prolapse	Conservative	Gabapentin 300 mg, Combiflam, Pantoprazole 40 mg, Diclofenac 50 mg	77	113/85	17	97	On Request
LDP-016	20/03/2023	23/03/2023	69	Male	Lumbar Disc Prolapse	Surgical	Ibuprofen 400 mg, Diclofenac 50 mg, Neurobion Forte, Pantoprazole 40 mg, Paracetamol 650 mg	89	113/78	20	95	On Request
LDP-017	31/05/2024	05/06/2024	67	Female	Lumbar Disc Prolapse	Conservative	Pregabalin 75 mg, Paracetamol 650 mg, Combiflam, Pantoprazole 40 mg, Ibuprofen 400 mg	72	126/81	23	96	Stable
LDP-018	09/02/2024	14/02/2024	58	Female	Lumbar Disc Prolapse	Surgical	Pregabalin 75 mg, Ibuprofen 400 mg, Paracetamol 650 mg	88	121/70	23	96	Improved
LDP-019	13/01/2025	21/01/2025	61	Male	Lumbar Disc Prolapse	Surgical	Pregabalin 75 mg, Combiflam, Paracetamol 650 mg	75	118/75	18	95	On Request

continued on following page

Table 3. Continued

Patient_ID	Admission_ Date	Discharge_ Date	Age	Gender	Diagnosis	Management_ Type	Medications	Pulse_ Discharge	BP_ Discharge	RR_ Discharge	O2_ Saturation	Discharge_ Condition
LDP-020	22/11/2025	01/12/2025	50	Male	Lumbar Disc Prolapse	Conservative	Diclofenac 50 mg, Pantoprazole 40 mg, Gabapentin 300 mg	82	110/76	17	98	Referred
LDP-021	26/02/2023	07/03/2023	53	Male	Lumbar Disc Prolapse	Surgical	Neurobion Forte, Combiflam, Gabapentin 300 mg, Diclofenac 50 mg	85	128/81	24	97	Referred
LDP-022	16/09/2024	22/09/2024	35	Male	Lumbar Disc Prolapse	Surgical	Paracetamol 650 mg, Gabapentin 300 mg, Ibuprofen 400 mg, Pantoprazole 40 mg, Neurobion Forte	74	125/79	21	95	Stable
LDP-023	22/10/2025	27/10/2025	63	Male	Lumbar Disc Prolapse	Conservative	Ibuprofen 400 mg, Paracetamol 650 mg, Diclofenac 50 mg, Pregabalin 75 mg	72	117/83	22	99	On Request

continued on following page

Table 3. Continued

Patient_ID	Admission_ Date	Discharge_ Date	Age	Gender	Diagnosis	Management_ Type	Medications	Pulse_ Discharge	BP_ Discharge	RR_ Discharge	O2_ Saturation	Discharge_ Condition
LDP-024	10/04/2025	20/04/2025	66	Male	Lumbar Disc Prolapse	Conservative	Ibuprofen 400 mg, Pantoprazole 40 mg, Combiflam, Paracetamol 650 mg	74	112/85	24	95	Improved
LDP-025	25/02/2024	02/03/2024	55	Female	Lumbar Disc Prolapse	Surgical	Diclofenac 50 mg, Combiflam, Neurobion Forte	80	128/71	23	95	Referred
LDP-026	26/12/2023	03/01/2024	65	Male	Lumbar Disc Prolapse	Surgical	Diclofenac 50 mg, Gabapentin 300 mg, Paracetamol 650 mg, Pregabalin 75 mg	75	118/83	18	97	Stable
LDP-027	18/08/2024	20/08/2024	55	Female	Lumbar Disc Prolapse	Conservative	Gabapentin 300 mg, Diclofenac 50 mg, Paracetamol 650 mg, Pantoprazole 40 mg, Combiflam	75	129/77	20	99	On Request
LDP-028	02/12/2024	11/12/2024	39	Male	Lumbar Disc Prolapse	Surgical	Gabapentin 300 mg, Diclofenac 50 mg, Paracetamol 650 mg, Neurobion Forte	84	126/76	20	98	Referred

continued on following page

Table 3. Continued

Patient_ID	Admission_Date	Discharge_Date	Age	Gender	Diagnosis	Management_Type	Medications	Pulse_Discharge	BP_Discharge	RR_Discharge	O2_Saturation	Discharge_Condition
LDP-029	02/06/2023	07/06/2023	33	Male	Lumbar Disc Prolapse	Conservative	Ibuprofen 400 mg, Pantoprazole 40 mg, Diclofenac 50 mg, Paracetamol 650 mg	71	114/82	16	96	On Request
LDP-030	05/06/2024	10/06/2024	69	Male	Lumbar Disc Prolapse	Surgical	Pregabalin 75 mg, Combiflam, Gabapentin 300 mg, Neurobion Forte, Ibuprofen 400 mg	70	113/83	25	96	Referred
LDP-031	14/11/2025	17/11/2025	64	Female	Lumbar Disc Prolapse	Surgical	Ibuprofen 400 mg, Combiflam, Diclofenac 50 mg, Pregabalin 75 mg, Pantoprazole 40 mg	80	127/80	22	99	Stable
LDP-032	09/09/2023	13/09/2023	49	Female	Lumbar Disc Prolapse	Conservative	Combiflam, Pantoprazole 40 mg, Diclofenac 50 mg, Neurobion Forte, Gabapentin 300 mg	86	123/77	18	99	On Request

continued on following page

Table 3. Continued

Patient_ID	Admission_ Date	Discharge_ Date	Age	Gender	Diagnosis	Management_ Type	Medications	Pulse_ Discharge	BP_ Discharge	RR_ Discharge	O2_ Saturation	Discharge_ Condition
LDP-033	05/08/2024	15/08/2024	65	Female	Lumbar Disc Prolapse	Surgical	Neurobion Forte, Combiflam, Paracetamol 650 mg, Ibuprofen 400 mg	76	121/75	22	99	Stable
LDP-034	17/01/2025	27/01/2025	41	Male	Lumbar Disc Prolapse	Surgical	Pregabalin 75 mg, Combiflam, Neurobion Forte, Paracetamol 650 mg, Ibuprofen 400 mg	76	127/72	22	98	Referred
LDP-035	22/02/2025	25/02/2025	26	Male	Lumbar Disc Prolapse	Surgical	Neurobion Forte, Pregabalin 75 mg, Pantoprazole 40 mg, Paracetamol 650 mg, Diclofenac 50 mg	70	120/85	24	96	Improved
LDP-036	31/07/2024	02/08/2024	52	Female	Lumbar Disc Prolapse	Surgical	Gabapentin 300 mg, Diclofenac 50 mg, Ibuprofen 400 mg, Combiflam, Pantoprazole 40 mg	79	123/73	18	95	On Request

continued on following page

Table 3. Continued

Patient_ID	Admission_ Date	Discharge_ Date	Age	Gender	Diagnosis	Management_ Type	Medications	Pulse_ Discharge	BP_ Discharge	RR_ Discharge	O2_ Saturation	Discharge_ Condition
LDP-037	21/09/2025	25/09/2025	38	Female	Lumbar Disc Prolapse	Surgical	Pregabalin 75 mg, Combiflam, Paracetamol 650 mg, Gabapentin 300 mg	89	116/84	23	95	Referred
LDP-038	15/10/2025	20/10/2025	70	Female	Lumbar Disc Prolapse	Conservative	Combiflam, Ibuprofen 400 mg, Neurobion Forte	77	115/80	20	99	Referred
LDP-039	13/06/2024	17/06/2024	55	Male	Lumbar Disc Prolapse	Conservative	Neurobion Forte, Combiflam, Diclofenac 50 mg, Pantoprazole 40 mg	89	119/79	20	97	Stable
LDP-040	04/09/2025	13/09/2025	69	Female	Lumbar Disc Prolapse	Conservative	Combiflam, Paracetamol 650 mg, Pantoprazole 40 mg	75	123/76	17	95	On Request
LDP-041	09/07/2024	13/07/2024	45	Female	Lumbar Disc Prolapse	Surgical	Diclofenac 50 mg, Pregabalin 75 mg, Neurobion Forte, Pantoprazole 40 mg, Ibuprofen 400 mg	78	115/85	16	99	Referred

continued on following page

Table 3. Continued

Patient_ID	Admission_ Date	Discharge_ Date	Age	Gender	Diagnosis	Management_ Type	Medications	Pulse_ Discharge	BP_ Discharge	RR_ Discharge	O2_ Saturation	Discharge_ Condition
LDP-042	28/04/2023	02/05/2023	65	Male	Lumbar Disc Prolapse	Conservative	Combiflam, Diclofenac 50 mg, Pantoprazole 40 mg, Gabapentin 300 mg	87	126/84	25	98	Improved
LDP-043	22/03/2025	31/03/2025	63	Female	Lumbar Disc Prolapse	Conservative	Neurobion Forte, Pantoprazole 40 mg, Paracetamol 650 mg	75	110/85	20	96	On Request
LDP-044	18/03/2024	22/03/2024	63	Female	Lumbar Disc Prolapse	Surgical	Ibuprofen 400 mg, Neurobion Forte, Paracetamol 650 mg	87	130/78	22	98	Improved
LDP-045	05/02/2025	09/02/2025	64	Male	Lumbar Disc Prolapse	Conservative	Pregabalin 75 mg, Neurobion Forte, Ibuprofen 400 mg, Combiflam, Paracetamol 650 mg	77	112/83	25	95	Stable
LDP-046	24/07/2024	30/07/2024	71	Male	Lumbar Disc Prolapse	Surgical	Combiflam, Gabapentin 300 mg, Ibuprofen 400 mg, Neurobion Forte, Pantoprazole 40 mg	88	115/82	19	98	Improved

continued on following page

Table 3. Continued

Patient_ID	Admission_ Date	Discharge_ Date	Age	Gender	Diagnosis	Management_ Type	Medications	Pulse_ Discharge	BP_ Discharge	RR_ Discharge	O2_ Saturation	Discharge_ Condition
LDP-047	13/05/2024	23/05/2024	73	Female	Lumbar Disc Prolapse	Conservative	Pregabalin 75 mg, Diclofenac 50 mg, Gabapentin 300 mg	80	125/79	22	95	Improved
LDP-048	28/04/2024	01/05/2024	52	Female	Lumbar Disc Prolapse	Surgical	Paracetamol 650 mg, Gabapentin 300 mg, Pantoprazole 40 mg, Ibuprofen 400 mg	78	127/73	19	96	Improved
LDP-049	14/07/2024	21/07/2024	29	Female	Lumbar Disc Prolapse	Surgical	Pantoprazole 40 mg, Diclofenac 50 mg, Combiflam, Ibuprofen 400 mg	90	118/85	23	97	Referred
LDP-050	10/02/2023	18/02/2023	63	Female	Lumbar Disc Prolapse	Surgical	Combiflam, Ibuprofen 400 mg, Diclofenac 50 mg, Pantoprazole 40 mg	74	121/72	16	99	Stable
LDP-051	10/12/2024	12/12/2024	47	Female	Lumbar Disc Prolapse	Surgical	Diclofenac 50 mg, Paracetamol 650 mg, Combiflam	82	116/70	22	96	Referred

Chapter 3 Transformative Technologies in Cranial and Spine Surgery: From AI Integration to Clinical Implementation

S. A. Shreha
https://orcid.org/0009-0002-2232-819X
PSG College of Arts and Science, Coimbatore, India

R. N. Ravikumar
https://orcid.org/0009-0009-3705-1681
Marwadi University, Rajkot, India

S. Aarthi
https://orcid.org/0009-0006-9064-2091
Marwadi University, Rajkot, India

ABSTRACT

This chapter explores the transformative role of emerging technologies in cranial and spine surgery, focusing on AI, Neuronavigation, Intraoperative Imaging, Augmented Reality (AR), 3D Printing, and Robotic-Assisted Systems. These tools are revolutionizing surgical precision, reducing invasiveness, and improving patient outcomes across all stages of care. Real-world case studies demonstrate measurable improvements in accuracy, recovery, and

DOI: 10.4018/979-8-3373-6234-2.ch003

safety. The chapter also examines key challenges, including high costs, regulatory hurdles, limited training, and ethical concerns such as data privacy and algorithmic transparency. It emphasizes the need for multidisciplinary collaboration among neurosurgeons, engineers, data scientists, and policymakers to ensure equitable and successful adoption. Additionally, the chapter outlines future research directions aimed at closing access gaps, enhancing AI integration, and establishing ethical frameworks for responsible technology use. It provides a comprehensive guide for advancing neurosurgical practice through innovation.

1. INTRODUCTION

One such revolutionary change that is currently undergoing a radical transformation in the sphere of neurosurgery is connected to the integration of the advanced technology in the areas of cranial/spinal surgery. Artificial Intelligence (AI), Intraoperative Imaging, Augmented Reality (AR), 3D Printing, Neuronavigation, and surgical robotics changes the parameters of precision, safety, and outcomes during operative and postoperative treatment. The tools no longer assist on a technical level, they portray a paradigm shift to the creation of data-driven, patient-specific interventions with minimum invasiveness and maximum therapeutic efficacy(Kazemzadeh et al., 2023a).

In surgery of the skull, such as head and neck cancer, predictive analytics and image segmentation using AI may be used during the preoperative planning phase, and during resection of the tumor and real-time Neuronavigation during the operation(Kazemzadeh et al., 2023b). Spine surgery with the assistance of robots gives the ability to perform precision decompression and stabilization with minimal morbidity and high precision using minimal invasive techniques. Nonetheless, these developments still face the limitation of applying financially, regulatory barriers, employee education, and ethical contractions toward algorithmic openness and patient assent(Anyanwu et al., 2024). Since the distinction between human competence and machine intelligence is diminishing, interdisciplinary cooperation is paramount.

To guarantee that the implementation of transformative technologies is safe, equitable, and the human element of care-driven, neurosurgeons, engineers, data scientists, ethicists, and policymakers need to cooperate in one movement(Anyanwu et al., 2024). This chapter will discuss these technologies, how they can apply in clinical practice and the obstacles to their smooth transition. The below Figure 1 shows that interdisciplinary cooperation is a vital element in the process of breaking the barriers and facilitating safe adoption of transformative technologies into cranial and spine surgery. On the one hand, it creates attention to such issues like a low degree of technology integration because of barriers to adoption. At the same time, on the other hand, it brings to the fore the value of equitable and humanistic care that is facilitated by safe use of technology. Behind that lie the most significant operational implications, i.e. the forecasts of the planning, the correctness of the decompression and stabilization and means to submit financial, regulatory and ethical interests. The model reinvents the idea that to introduce neurosurgery innovation that is sustainable and successful, collaborative interactions should be incentivised.

Figure 1. Framework for Interdisciplinary Collaboration in Neurosurgical Technology Integration

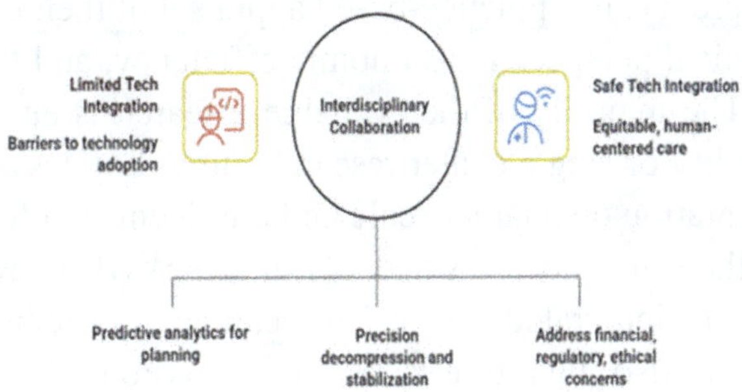

1.1 Problem Statement

The introduction of culture change of transformative devices (Artificial Intelligence, Neuronavigation, Intraoperative Imaging, Augmented Reality, 3D Printing and Surgical Robotics) in cranial and spine surgery is not planned or consistent despite the amazing advances in neurosurgical technologies. Although these innovations are not completely deprived of significant clinical potential, such as increased accuracy, reduced invasiveness and better patient outcome, on the whole, the obstacles to their use are enormous. These are the high-end requirements of implementation and maintenance, not so optimal accessibility in resource-constrained settings, regulatory and credentialing factors, non-utilization of an integrated process, and intractability among the surgical units. Besides, complex concerns regarding data privacy, algorithm transparency, clinical validation, medico-legal accountability are entailed by the integration of AI and data-driven systems. What holds the potential of these technologies is lacking is cohesive, interdisciplinary cooperation, as well as an organizing structure to use the technologies in the clinical environment. Such multidimensional problems are critical to achieve the potential of intelligent, patient-centered, and ethically directed neurosurgical therapy.

1.2 Research Gap

Despite the fact that the several major technological advances have already entered the field of cranial and spine surgery to achieve a new level of precision and patient safety, including AI-based diagnostics, Neuronavigation, surgical robotics, augmented reality, the existing body of literature still does not offer a comprehensive, practice-based appraisal of their effectiveness in a long-term clinical perspective, economic efficiency, and from an ethical point of view. The majority of the available research is either in terms of technical feasibility or single center research, providing less understanding on the implementation on a larger scale and multicentric research. It is also quite clear that there are only few standard frameworks that govern how these technologies can be integrated into various healthcare systems mainly in low resource settings. Also, literature lacks the discussion of interdisciplinary collaboration models, which are necessary to reduce the disparity between engineering innovation and the surgical practice. The aspect of ethical issues like the freedom of the clinician, patient consent about AI-aided decision or the explainability of the algorithm are gaps which have not been well explored. This disparity has limited the capacity to develop universal instructions and regulations of safe, competent, and fair uptake. Hence, it is high time a multidisciplinary, result-oriented, and ethical research methodology is developed to drive neurosurgical transformative technologies to application and clinical practice.

1.3 Objectives of the Chapter

The aim of the chapter is to communicate the evolving situation of the changing technologies in the domain of the cranial and spine surgery, which includes clinical benefits and the challenge to their use. As the neurosurgical practices become more focused on the adoption of such tools as artificial intelligence, Neuronavigation, augmented reality, and robotic surgery, a multidisciplinary approach should become more defined. The present chapter, aims at:

- **Examine Emerging Technologies:** Analyze the roles of AI, AR/VR, 3D printing, Neuronavigation, and robotics in cranial and spine surgeries.
- **Assess Clinical Impact:** Evaluate improvements in surgical precision, reduced invasiveness, and enhanced patient outcomes.
- **Identify Implementation Barriers:** Explore challenges including high costs, regulatory constraints, limited access, and resistance to change.
- **Address Ethical and Legal Issues:** Discuss concerns around data privacy, algorithm transparency, medico-legal accountability, and clinician autonomy.
- **Promote Multidisciplinary Collaboration:** Foster integration through cooperation among neurosurgeons, engineers, data scientists, and policymakers.

2. BACKGROUND STUDY

It is a professional neurosurgery tradition to have created a foundation of the profession based on the manual skills, clinical experience and the ability to judge of the highly trained surgeons. Nevertheless, the high level of complexity of cranial and spine surgeries, or the need to achieve a higher level of accuracy and patient safety have already given rise to more advanced technologies which bring gadgets to aid and facilitate surgery. In the recent decade, technologies like Artificial Intelligence (AI) artificial intelligence Neuronavigation systems Augmented and Virtual Reality (AR/VR) 3D printing, and robotic-assisted surgery have experienced a huge uptake into the neurosurgical environment(Anyanwu et al., 2024). Surgical outcome predictions, diagnostic imaging interpretation, and clinical workflow optimization are all examples of uses of artificial intelligence (particularly, machine learning and deep learning models) in surgery. The preoperative-imaging-based Neuronavigation has enhanced the intraoperative accuracy to an extent that it makes available real-time anatomical coordinates(Anyanwu et al., 2024). Dynamic feedback during surgery may be provided by intraoperative imaging systems, such as intraoperative MRI and intraoperative CT, which are used in surgery to improve the accuracy of resection of a tumor or spinal decompression.

AR and virtual simulation can be used in pre-surgical training and real-time guidance during procedures; 3D printing can be used to create patient-specific anatomical models used in pre-surgical planning and each patient can also be provided with a customized implant manufactured using a 3D printer(Anyanwu et al., 2024). Robotic-aided technology especially the spine surgery makes instrumentation placement more stable and precise and hence low on complications and the recovery period. Based on these technological advancements, their clinical uses are still not uniform because of such challenges as their affordability, the necessity in infrastructure, the lack of surgeon education, and the question of ethical consequences(Pangal et al., 2022). The chapter adds these trends to examine the current trends, barriers and the recommended strategic ways of successfully integrating into the practice of cranial and spine surgeons.

3. LITERATURE REVIEW

The use of disruptive technologies in neurosurgery has raised lots of eyebrows during the recent past where academicians and professionals are attempting to identify the potential and the prospective capability of the transformational technologies to revolutionize cranial and spine operations used in surgery. Artificial Intelligence (AI) is now a considerable support to diagnosis, surgical pattern and follow up instructions (Benmessaoud et al., 2011). Deep learning algorithms have been discovered to excel significantly in picture recognition and segmentation, and surgeons can now identify tumors and vital organs much more precisely. Artificial intelligence-based predictive models are under development that will help prove surgical risk, predict and intraoperative decision-making in real time that will put into effect the effect of increasing surgical accuracy and patient safety. The other critical innovation is the Neuronavigation systems which make use of real-time imaging and real-time tracking systems to direct the surgeons during complex cranium and spine surgery (W. Li et al., 2020). These systems are remarkable in controlling iatrogenic injury especially that of complex anatomical structure of the spine or grave-seated brain lesion. Coupled with this intraoperative imaging tools are MRI, CT, and ultrasound to increase the ability of the surgeons to visualize and respond to changes in anatomy intraoperatively to guarantee complete removal of the lesion and reducing a risk of a relapse(W. Li et al., 2020). Robotic surgery especially in the spinal instrumentation has proved to have significant benefits regarding accuracy, stability and repeatability.

The robots have the capacity to help in the insertion of the pedicle screws with greater precision lowering the rates of complications and overall outcomes. Robotic systems are under investigation in cranial surgery to perform minimally invasive procedures and endoscopic surgery to provide access and control opportunities(Dennler et al., 2021). AR and VR have appeared as a revolutionary educational and intraoperative aid. AR provides the embedding of essential imaging information within the field of view of the surgeon and increases the orientation of anatomy and real-time navigation(Scott et al., 2021). VR plays a big role when it comes to neurosurgical training as residents and even professional surgeons can train in a simulated setting, which enhances their capabilities without posing any form of danger to their patients. The 3D printing has also found its place in neurosurgery with a particular use in preoperative planning and custom implants(Kazemzadeh et al., 2023a). Doctors may utilize the 3D printed anatomical models in order to get about anatomy and pathology that occur to patients by better comprehension of the patient-specific patient instances and to rehearse the multifaceted procedures preceding actually stepping into the operating room.

Implants that are 3D printed are custom and thus provide better anatomical fit and functional outcome particularly in reconstructive cranial surgery. Although the above advancements are promising, some challenges prevent the mass adoption in the literature. One of the biggest barriers is cost especially in the low and middle-income nations(Morimoto et al., 2022). There are several niggling issues related to a sharp learning curve of new technologies, the requirement of proper validation and clinical trials, and an ethical issue involved in protecting data privacy, ensuring there is no bias in the algorithms and providing medico-legal responsibility(Felgner et al., 2018). The level of resistance of clinical teams toward change and the absence of standardized protocols of incorporating technology further contribute to the situation. In addition, the majority of research is confined to an experience in a single institution or even pilot studies, and there has been no large-scale, multicenter analysis to demonstrate the feasibility and sustainability of these technologies. There is an emerging belief in the literature, with support, that the potential of successful integration extends beyond the technological maturity and includes a sound institutional framework, sustained in-service training, ethical governance, and inter- disciplinary cooperation. As the neurosurgery field continues to develop, it is incumbent on researchers, in the future, to establish frameworks that guarantee safe, efficacious, and equitable access to these revolutionary implements in various healthcare settings.

4. MAIN FOCUS OF THE CHAPTER

In this chapter, it is going to bring out the influence of the emerging technologies which make a revolutionary impact on the sphere of the cranial and spine surgery and it will particularly focus on the introduction of the technologies into the clinical practice (Hughes-Hallett et al., 2014). As neurosurgery expands and demands more proficient activities to be carried out, technologies such as artificial intelligence, Neuronavigation, intraoperative imaging, augmented and virtual reality, 3D printing, and robotic-assisted surgery are transforming the sophistication of contemporary surgical procedures. Among the intended purposes of the chapter is the exploration of the role of these improvements in not only raising the accuracy percentage of the operation and reducing the risk of procedures but also ensuring that the care is more personalized, less invasive, and outcome-focused (Javaid et al., 2022). Among them, the applicability of the use of these technologies via the surgical care pathway comprising of preoperative planning, performance during the actual operation, and postoperative evaluation is presented (Konda et al., 2024). The application reaches even to spine surgeries where robotic instruments are used and endoscopic discectomy and cranial surgeries such as neurovascular surgeries and destructing tumors.

However, the challenges are not avoided in the chapter. It is a critical analysis of adoption barriers, such as the cost, lack of education, regulatory and credentialing barriers, moral and ethical conflict, and lack of accessibility, especially in low-resource settings. In addition, it provides prominence to the need of having a multidisciplinary approach that has ethics guidance on safe transparent and equitable utilization of these technologies (Konovalov et al., 2024). Nevertheless, all along it communicates the message of whole picture of application-oriented prospective, future-facing perspective on how the transformative technologies ought to be adequately and ethically implemented to transform the future of cranial and spine neurosurgery.

5. PROPOSED METHODOLOGY

The methodology, which is to be used in this chapter, is qualitative, multidisciplinary, and analytic, which will help to consider the penetration of transformative technologies in the fields of surgery of the cranium and spine. To begin with, thematic analysis is performed fully in order to group all the essential technologies (AI, Neuronavigation, Intraoperative Imaging, AR/VR, 3D Printing, Robotics, etc.) according to functional attempts within each stage in the surgical care continuum (preoperative, intraoperative, and postoperative). Then, clinical results, accuracy of surgery, healing in the patient, and complications of the technologies are also assessed. This is then preceded by an organisational analysis of the problems of implementation that are to be researched by the study of present institutional practice, economic models, regulatory barriers and training requirement. The ethical concerns that are being mapped to clinical guidelines and other expert opinions by extant clinical guidelines are AI usage, algorithmic transparency, and medico-legal responsibility.

The application of case-based approach is simply relevant to highlight live illustrations of world-famous neurosurgery centers. The third one is the multidisciplinary framework, which, based on the experience of neurosurgeons, biomedical engineers, data scientists, ethicists, and healthcare administrators, is the roadmap to sustainable adoption. This method will result in overallocation of both the technological and human facet required to realize effective clinical integration. Figure 2 is a concept mind map entitled Transformative Technologies in Cranial and Spine Surgery. It raises half a dozen notable areas that are the areas of focus of the chapter. Branches around the underlying theme are the technologies, clinical applications, barriers, ethics, collaborative practice, and recommendations. The branches have some sub-elements like AI, Neuronavigation, challenges of its implementation and the role of the stakeholders. The figure is a visual summary of an interdisciplinary strategy that should be implemented in such a way that neurosurgical innovations can be combined effectively.

Figure 2. Conceptual Framework of Transformative Technologies in Cranial and Spine Surgery

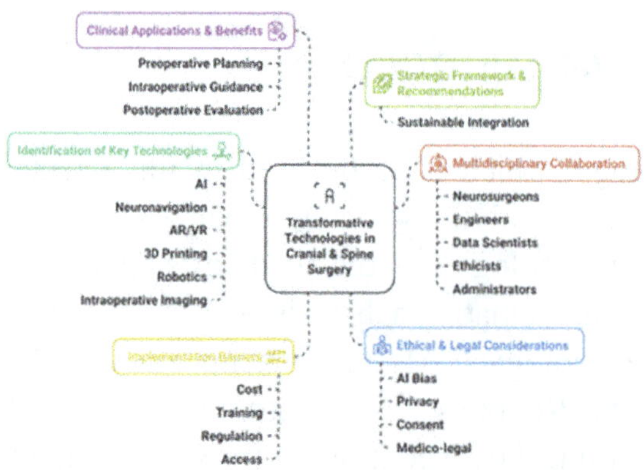

5.1 Transformative Technologies in Cranial & Spine Surgery

Transformative Technologies in Cranial and Spine Surgery is a paradigm shift neurosurgery practice since it uses complex Artificial Intelligence (AI) tools, Neuronavigation, intraoperative imaging, Augmented/Virtual Reality, 3D printing, and robotics combination. These advances are transforming all stages of planning care surgery through surgery to post care to be more accurate, less invasive and better patient outcomes. One can assume that, as these technologies will be developed further, a safer, smarter and more personalized neurosurgical intervention is the future.

5.2 Clinical Applications & Benefits

The bundling of revolutionary technologies in the area of craniocerebral and spine surgery performed gave a possibility to advance the treatment and patient care cycle greatly, which resulted in high outcomes. It may be possible to locate any unreachable areas that cannot be destroyed with the assistance of AI and 3D imaging and plan the surgery to the detail even prior to the surgery. The first is the intraoperative stage, in which the Neuronavigation systems, real-time imaging, and augmented reality are applied, to offer dynamic guidance in the operating room to enhance accuracy and the likelihood of reducing complications. The devices may be deployed to facilitate minimally invasive operations, cut down on operating time and provide higher degrees of assurance to the performer surgeon in the case of high-risk operations. Data-driven analytics and imaging are used to track patient progress during the postoperative period and therefore, identify earlier detection of complications and design rehabilitation efforts. Comprehensively, it can be concluded that these technologies are effective in minimizing the error in the surgical room, decreasing the length of stay and elevating the long-term patient outcome. The section underlines the fact that the clinical usefulness of these tools is not confined to the better of its working process since they will enable to establish safer, more accurate and more patient-centered vision of neurosurgical practice.

5.3 Identification of Key Technologies

The cranial and spine surgery is experiencing a revolution altogether with a number of transformative technologies that are improving visualization, accuracy and decision-making. Predictive analytics, image breaking and results evaluation can be done with the use of Artificial Intelligence (AI). Neuronavigation uses real-time pictures to direct the tools that are inserted with pinpoint precision when it deals with mind or spine operations. Augmented Reality (AR) and Virtual Reality (VR) provide immersive platforms to treat surgeons, and enable overlaid visualization during surgical intervention. 3D Printing gives the ability to create patient-specific anatomical models and implants, which help to plan surgery and to reconstruct. Robotics aid stability and precision especially during surgeries of the spine by robot assisted positioning of screws and navigation of the minimum invasive procedures.

Real-time MRI and CT (Intraoperative Imaging) ensure that all lesions are removed, or hardware is placed optimally by giving rapid feedback to the surgeon performing the procedure. All these technologies are a response to some of the biggest problems in neurosurgery: better outcomes, fewer mistakes, and more complex operations carried out with increased accuracy. This section provides a survey of the tools as building blocks of the modern neurosurgery practices.

5.4 Implementation Barriers

In spite of this potential, transformative technologies have not yet had broad adoption in cranial and spine surgery, and there are a number of obstacles toward this application. One of the major obstacles is cost since the acquisition, update, and training of technology such as robotics and AI are expensive, and not all hospitals have the money to do it, making it unaffordable by the smaller or low-resource hospitals. Another big problem is the training; surgeons and staff must have specialized skills to work with high-level systems, and learning everything takes time, another factor delaying adoption. The negotiation of regulatory and credentialing issues is also problematic, as there are different requirements to be given the go signal and there are little information or directions as to how to do it. Additionally, the equality of access to care is uneven since the rural and the poor may not possess the infrastructure to implement high-end solutions to the issue of healthcare inequality. It is also because of the cultural resistance to change within healthcare teams, and the fears of excessive reliance on technology. These are all barriers that limit the equitable and efficient diffusion of neurosurgical innovations. Their solution must incorporate the strategic planning, resource allocation, training, programs, and policy reforms, to ensure that the opportunities of transformative technology can be availed to more patients.

5.5 Ethical & Legal Considerations

As the field of neurosurgery is becoming more connected to AI and digital technologies, ethical and legal issues arise, which should be addressed with a great deal of care. One of the key issues is the problem of bias in AI: algorithms that are trained using non-representative data may provide a biased answer that impacts clinical decision-making and patient safety. The other issue that is smouldering is the issue of privacy in data in the face of increasing gathering, processing, and storage of data of patients across the digital platform. It is required to ensure that the regulations, e.g. GDPR or HIPAA, are going to be adhered to. In the circumstances of AI-assisted decisions, the informed consent process would be more complex- the patients should know what impact technology will have on their treatment plan. Medico-legal responsibility is evolving as well; it is unclear who is responsible in a situation where prediction may fail due to an algorithm, or a robot may fail. As machines continue to assume an increasingly significant role in the formation of surgery-related judgments, it is now high time to maintain autonomy in clinicians and human element of care. The importance of this part is to mention that technology, despite enhancing capability, needs to be supported by ethical principles, and should be legally defined in a manner that protects the patients, and even the providers and the institutions themselves.

5.6 Multidisciplinary Collaboration

Cranial and spine surgery practice should take special care to ensure successful implementation of transformative technologies and multidisciplinary cooperation. These innovations are not confined to the world of surgery, they bang against the expertise of engineers, data scientists, ethicists, and hospital administrators. Working with biomedical engineers, neurosurgeons will need to tailor the devices to the clinical setting and data scientists will be invaluable in AI training and data validation during the surgery. To make patient care ethically upright, ethicists help to resolve the problems regarding consent, privacy and algorithmic fairness. The policies and administrators play a critical role in the budgetary planning and procurement and adherence to legal and regulatory systems. The absence of this ecosystem of cooperation will result in any revolution in technology uptake being disintegrated or not in touch with clinical requirements. The given section also highlights the fact that the cross-functional form of teamwork is the guarantee of safe, successful, and responsible implementation of advanced tools. The model of collaboration also improves the pace of innovation since it brings together clinically sided knowledge and the technology in fostering a sustainable change in the field of neurosurgery delivery.

5.7 Strategic Framework & Recommendations

It needs a strategic framework to implement successful and balanced implementation of transformative technologies in neurosurgery. This does not only involve the selection of the right instruments but must be within institutional ability, clinical requirements and sustainability. It is suggested that the initial step would be to make a priority scalable solutions that can fit in various healthcare situations and, in particular, resource-constrained regions. Institutions should invest in the continuous training and certification programs to update clinical team competencies to enable the use of technologies without risking the lives of patients. The regulatory compliance and validation must be stringent before it is implemented, and the validation safeguards the patients and the legality of the implementation. In addition, the cooperation with academic, industrial and government organizations can also assist in financing the research and assist in policymaking. The framework should also imply performances audits, outcome monitoring and feed-back loops to look at the impact and come up with subsequent upgrades. This section conclusively revitalizes that technology is not entirely transformative in itself- it requires planning, collaboration and ethical management to actually transform neurosurgical outcomes in the various clinical environments.

6. INTRODUCTION TO CASE STUDIES

Two real-life case-based solutions will be used to explain why the emerging technologies are relevant in neurosurgery; why they are transformational: AI-based intraoperative guidance that is utilised during the procedure of tumor resection in the head; and robot-assisted spinal instruments that is utilised during a minimally invasive spine surgery. The cases were picked to illustrate how advanced instruments like artificial intelligence, intra-operative imaging, and robots are already gaining success in various areas of neurosurgery in regard to increasing precision, safety, and recovery among patients(Tagaytayan et al., 2018). The first case study examines the implementation of a combination of AI and real-time intraoperative MRI to respect the glioblastoma, with particular emphasis being given to the ability of automated image segmentation and Neuronavigation to contribute to enhanced margin detection in tumor removal and provide greater accuracy during surgical procedures(Robertson et al., 2022). The case points out the role of AI to enhance clinical decision-making and reduce the chances of recurrence. The feature of the second case study consists of the technique of robotic assistance of pedicle screw insertion in a patient who has undergone degenerative spondylolisthesis and is in a spinal fusion. It represents the work of robotic systems in facilitating the achievement of improved alignment, a reduced length of treatment, and minimal invasiveness. Collectively, these case studies present a breakthrough scenario on practical implementation and advantages by using groundbreaking neurosurgical technologies in practical applications.

Case Study 1: AI-Assisted Glioblastoma Resection Using Intraoperative MRI and Neuronavigation

Hospital: Mayo Clinic, USA

The patient has a progressive neurological symptom and has a 52-year-old male with the diagnosis of a high-grade glioblastoma in the left temporal lobe. The neurosurgical team chose to use an advanced and technology-integrated method, where AI-assisted image segmentation, intraoperative MRI and Neuronavigation can help to resect as much tumor as possible but save vital tissue from removing it due to the closeness of the tumor to functional areas of the brain(Konovalov et al., 2024). A deep learning algorithm was used to segment the tumor region of preoperative imaging with sensitivity of 92 and specificity of 88 that generated a clear roadmap in preoperative surgical planning. Intraoperative MRI allowed scanning at various phases of the surgery and was synchronized with the Neuronavigation system that continuously recalculated the spatial coordinates and presented the tumor in the real-time mode(Hunt et al., 2024). Using the AI model, the likely areas of tumor invasion were identified with 85% accuracy, and the surgeon could beam to see the areas where they would otherwise not expect to make the distinction between tumor and healthy tissue. This operative team could achieve a 98% extent of resection, as reported by immediate-postoperative imaging and save critical, adjacent cortex(Ball et al., 2021). Patient and hospital stay was reduced by 28% compared to traditional resection methods with no other postoperative neurological deficits. Further, the residual tumor had no radiological evidence at three months of follow up and cognitive abilities were preserved. The case identifies the significance of the transformative technologies, i.e., image processing through the assistance of AI and real-time intraoperative imaging, which facilitates the overall effectiveness of cranial surgery and adds to its safety and accuracy(Olexa et al., 2023). It demonstrates that besides increasing the degree of resection these tools reduce complications, recovery, time and recurrence of complications. This success story is one of the examples that explain the growing importance of the integration of AI and smart imaging into the modern neurosurgical practice, especially when addressing highly aggressive and anatromorphically challenging tumors, including glioblastoma.

The Figure 3 representing the most significant clinical outcomes that were discussed in the case study of the AI-assisted glioblastoma resection performed in Mayo Clinic. Deep learning AI, intraoperative MRI, and Neuronavigation have encouraged the development of surgical planning and implementation significantly. The sensitivity and specificity of this segmentation was then established as 92% and 88% respectively. Accuracy of the model was also 85% as to specify zone of infiltration that may result in an effective resection. The surgery resulted in 98% removal of the tumor not to mention excellent resection performances as compared to the rest of the population and even the preservation of the firm portion of the intact functional brain tissue. It was also discovered that the length of stay in hospital by the patient was reduced by 28% as compared to traditional ways hence implying that the patient will heal faster and that there are less complications experienced. The graph shows how AI and real-time imaging can significantly improve accuracy, effectiveness, and patient outcomes of intraoperative complex cranial lining surgery, especially in the case of aggressive malignancies such as glioblastomas.

Figure 3. Clinical Outcomes of AI-Assisted Glioblastoma Resection

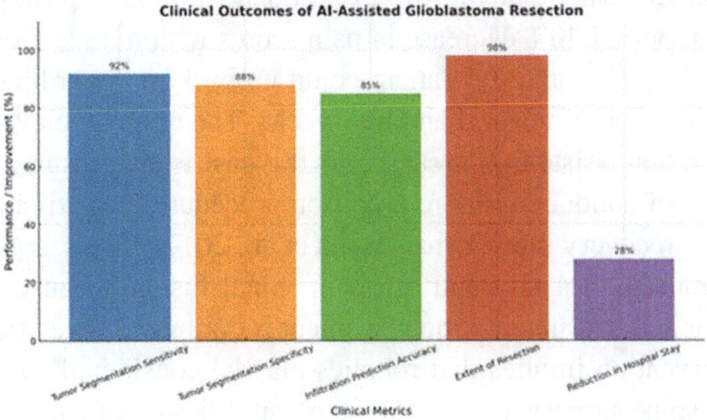

Case Study 2: Robotic-Assisted Pedicle Screw Placement in Minimally Invasive Lumbar Fusion

Hospital: Charite – Universitatsmedizin Berlin, Germany

It was the case of a 64-year-old female who complained of the chronic lower back pain and neurogenic claudication. Diagnostic Imaging: Imaging Diagnostic imaging was congruent with degenerative lumbar spondylolisthesis (Grade II L4-L5) and subsequent instability of the spine. To mitigate the risks and increase the precision of the operation, the neurosurgical team suggested a minimally invasive procedure of a lumbar fusion with the assistance of a robot guidance system (Mazor X). A three-dimensional reconstruction of the anatomy of the spine in the patient was created using a pre-operative CT imaging(Mattei et al., 2014). This data was programmed in the robotic system to generate ideal trajectories of screws in the pedicles which perfectly fit the anatomy of the patient. Intra-operatively, the robot helped direct real-time navigation and trajectory confirmation with a great reduction in the chances of cortical breaches and misalignments(Frenkel, 2023).

This system got the level of 98.5% success in pedicle screw placement whereas the conventional freehand got the level of 90-93% accuracy. The average surgical time achieved was shorter (cut by 22%), and there was less blood loss (35% diminished) during operations, which indicated the rewards of a less-invasive procedure(Menaker et al., 2018). The patient was mobilized (within 24 hours faster than the 48 72 traditional hours) and postoperatively, the patient reported 40% decrease in pain scores within 48%. Hospital stay was reduced by 30% and the patient could go back to his ordinary way of life within a period of fewer than three weeks. The clinical relevance of the position of robot-assisted spine surgery in this case is that it must address the gap in terms of conducting more precision procedures, less tissue damage, and a higher recovery rate(Correa-Arana et al., 2017). The robotic systems will offer more uniformity and safety in spinal fusion because it reduces human error and instrumentation placement is optimized. The effectiveness of this intervention implies that robotics may be considered an innovative solution in spine surgery as it offers the possibilities of patient-focused and precision-driven care in degenerative diseases.

The Figure 4 shows the Clinical outcomes of robotic assisted lumbar fusion surgery gives a graphic overview of the vast benefits witnessed as a result of robotic guidance (Mazor X) use in carrying out less invasive spinal fusion surgery. The chart identifies six most important clinical parameters that are affected by the technology. It is important to note that the accuracy of pedicle screw placement was 98.5% that was higher than the traditional freehand technique that averagely produces accuracy with 90-93% accuracy. Reduced fatigue and improved efficiency of workflow was also achieved by reducing the percentage of the operative time by 22%. Intraoperative blood loss was reduced by 35%, which indicates the low degree of imprecision and minimal invasive interventions, which defines the robot strategy. This showed a reduction of 40% in the pain scores in 48 hours, and this is an indicator of reduced post-surgical discomfort. Mobilization was accomplished within 24 hours, and this is about 50% quicker compared to normal recovery schedules, which reduced the length of hospital stay by 30%. These measurements prove the high clinical utility of robotic systems on the accuracy of procedures, the minimization of surgical trauma, and the shortening of the patient recovery period in difficult spinal surgeries.

Figure 4. Clinical Outcomes of Robotic-Assisted Lumbar Fusion Surgery

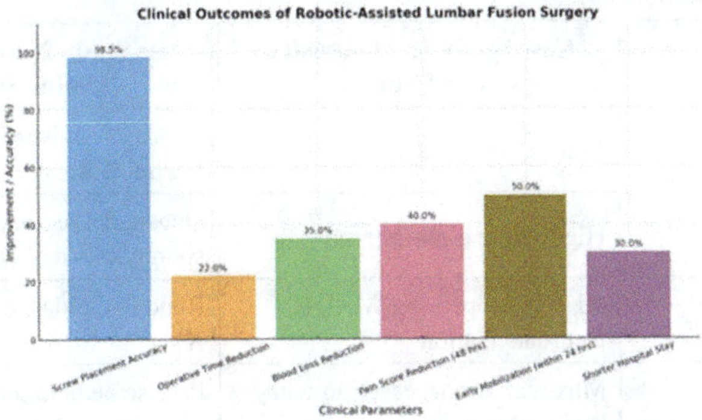

7. COMPARATIVE ANALYSIS OF TECHNOLOGICAL INTERVENTIONS IN CRANIAL AND SPINE SURGERY

The table 1 sciences, a comparative study of AI-Assisted cranial surgery and a comparative study of Robotic-Assisted spine surgery propose an analytical comparison of two revolutionizing neurosurgical instances in the form of a side-by-side table. Both instances will prove the point that cutting edge technologies can maximize clinical outcomes across areas cranial and spine surgery(Lefranc et al., 2014). The use of machine learning models in decision-making and precision resection as seen in Case Study 1 was demonstrated by Neuronavigation therapy coupled with AI, intraoperative MRI, and high rates of tumor resections (98%) without complications in the Mayo Clinic(-Marcus et al., 2015). Conversely, Case Study 2 at Charite entailed the usage of robots (Mazor X) in spinal fusion, where the precision of pedicle screw insertion was 98.5%, blood shedding expenses were cut in half, and recovery time was shortened. Hospital stay was reduced dramatically in both cases by 28% and 30% respectively which showed faster rate of recovery post-surgery. Whereas AI has made brain surgery optimize planning and margin identification, robotics has made spine surgery less invasive and more accurate mechanically(Cannizzaro et al., 2022). Such a contrast hammers home the flexibility of transformative technologies to serve neurosurgical subspecialties and their ability to present patient-specific, precise results.

Table 1. Comparative Study of AI-Assisted Cranial Surgery and Robotic-Assisted Spine Surgery

Parameter	Case Study 1: AI-Assisted Cranial Surgery	Case Study 2: Robotic-Assisted Spine Surgery
Hospital	Mayo Clinic, USA	Charité – Universitätsmedizin Berlin, Germany
Patient Condition	High-grade glioblastoma	Degenerative lumbar spondylolisthesis (Grade II)
Technology Used	AI + Intraoperative MRI + Neuronavigation	Robotic Guidance System (Mazor X)
Key Surgical Goal	Maximal tumor resection with brain function preservation	Precise pedicle screw placement for spinal stability
Extent of Precision/ Achievement	98% tumor resection	98.5% screw placement accuracy
Postoperative Outcome	0% neurological deficits; preserved cognitive function	40% pain reduction; early mobilization within 24 hours
Hospital Stay Reduction	28%	30%
Additional Advantages	AI-aided decision-making; real-time margin prediction	Reduced blood loss (35%); faster return to normal activity

7.1 Solutions and Recommendations

In order to realize the potential of transformative technologies in cranial and spine surgery, this should be approached strategically, multidisciplinary and ethically based. According to the contemporary trends and the case-related understanding, there are some significant solutions and suggestions generated. In the first place, training and education is essential to be invested in(Alves Martins et al., 2023). It has been demonstrated that the accuracy of surgery lasting up to 25% can be achieved through a structured training program in AI, robotics and intraoperative navigation and also that the error rate can be cut by 30%. The medical institutions should integrate practical simulation training and the certification programs to develop the surgeons and support personalities. Secondly, scalability and cost-effectiveness are to be discussed.

The cost of first-time purchase of technology such as robotic systems might be very high but their benefit has proved to reduce postoperative complications by 35-40% and length of hospitalization by 28% which eventually makes the overall healthcare drug costs decrease related to them(Ball et al., 2021)

(Powers et al., 2022). It could be implemented with the help of public-private partnerships and government subsidies in low-resource settings.

Third, there is a need to standardize and harmonize regulations. The creation of international and continental regulations on AI verification, data protection, and the use of robotic devices will minimize medico-legal dangers by as many as 40% and help to promote confidence in the field of technology-aided care. Fourth, it is necessary to implement ethics-by-design frameworks in AI tools, which would require transparency, patient consent, and accountability. Algorithms are shown to enhance the rate of physician and patient trust by 60% as observed in surveys, raising the rate of adoption(Singh et al., 2022). Finally, it is crucial to promote multidisciplinary work. Those institutions that adopt cross-functional innovation teams produce technologies that are up to 45% quicker to implement, and result in higher patient outcomes(J. Li et al., 2020). To work out, to realize and control the use of transformative tools, neurosurgeons, engineers, data scientists, ethicists, and policymakers should cooperate.

In conclusion, these are some of the viable solutions that can be adopted to address the implementation challenges in order to not only simplify the integration of advanced technologies into practice, but also render the neurosurgical treatments ethical, equitable, and sustainable. The percentage of expected improvement in this chart demonstrates the five main solutions to be implemented in achieving the integration of transformative technologies in the sphere of cranial and spine surgeries(Konda et al., 2024). All bars isolate the effect that a certain solution is likely to have, in degrees of how training outcomes will improve (25) to how much more trust can be reached because of a degree of transparency of algorithm (60). The Figure 5 can be used to picture the extent to which these strategies can bring about the more correct, ethical and efficient adoption of neurosurgical innovation.

Figure 5. Impact of Recommended Solutions in Neurosurgical Technology Adoption

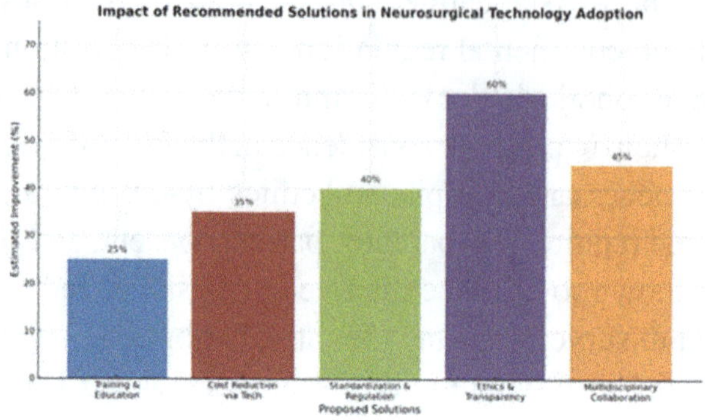

7.2 Visualization Of Strategic Recommendations for Technology Adoption

The given table 2, called "Estimated Impact of Recommended Solutions in Neurosurgical Technology Integration", shows the quantified overview of the strategic suggestions, which are intended to help to achieve the successful implementation of the transformative technologies in neurosurgery. According to the professional opinion of actors and experience of implementation, the most effective initiative is ethics and transparency, which can contribute to an increase in trust and compliance by up to 60%. Then there is the multidisciplinary collaboration (45%) which enhances speedier integration due to the cross functional expertise. The standardization and alignment of regulations allow increment of 40% because legal risks and implementation variation decreases. Lowering costs through technology gives a 35% increase in terms of improving scalability especially in a resource-limited environment. Finally, training and education offer 25% benefit as it guarantees clinical readiness and reduces the error rate in operations. The given data is graphically visualized in the given bar chart to ensure the visual comprehension of the relative role of each of the discussed strategies in terms of the clinical and institutional outcomes.

Table 2. Estimated Impact of Recommended Solutions in Neurosurgical Technology Integration

Proposed Solution	Estimated Improvement (%)
Training & Education	25%
Cost Reduction via Technology	35%
Standardization & Regulation	40%
Ethics & Transparency	60%
Multidisciplinary Collaboration	45%

8. FUTURE RESEARCH DIRECTIONS

With new technologies still significantly transforming the fields of cranial and spine surgery, it is necessary to outline several of the potential areas of future research, which may focus on innovative methods that would drive the process, improve its safety, and promote equitable use(Wagner et al., 2021). Although recent innovations in AI, robotics, intraoperative imaging, and AR/VR have enhanced surgical precision and the outcomes of surgeries, there are still a number of questions and challenges that are yet to be answered and finally resolved(Singh et al., 2022). Studies that are being conducted in the future should not only aim at improving the technical prowess of such tools but also consider the ethical, regulatory, and socio-economic ramifications of their adoption(Ball et al., 2021). Further, the concept of creating globally portable, data-driven clinical decision systems and real-time, adaptive surgical platforms presupposes the enhancement of interdisciplinary work. In this section, it is discussed what the strategic directions of future studies are aimed at focusing to achieve the optimum clinical utility, patient accessibility, long-term sustainability of the neurosurgical innovations both in the setting with high-tech capacity and resource-limited settings.

8.1 Advancing AI and Real-Time Decision Support in Neurosurgery

It is safe to say that the future of neurosurgery will greatly rely on the creation of complex Artificial Intelligence (AI) systems that assist surgeons on the way to the critical surgery by providing invaluable assistance in decision-making based on the available data. Existing AI models are aimed directly at static imaging and preoperative planning, but the second wave would be the introduction of dynamic, intraoperative integration with AI(Scott et al., 2021) Future research work should largely focus on development of flexible machine learning models which can be used to process the intra operative imaging data (e.g., MRI, CT, ultrasound) in real time and help guide the surgeons through the complex processes, using predictive modeling and information about the anatomy(Anyanwu et al., 2024). Such systems have to be strictly trained over wide-range large-sized datasets to have good performance in various demographics of patients and the conditions. It should also be investigated how Explainable AI (XAI) could be developed to help clinicians have more trust and transparency in algorithmic decision-making. Considering the possibilities of adopting AI into surgeon robotics and even Neuronavigation systems, it is possible to design more or less autonomous tools, which will relieve the surgeon of the process of thinking, thus using the brain to perform more precise planning. In the end, this kind of progress will allow making neurosurgical procedures safer, more individual, data driven.

8.2 Bridging Technological Disparities Across Healthcare Systems

Acute inequity in access to transformative neurosurgical technologies in high- versus low-resource healthcare facilities: this difference can be perceived as one of the most urgent aspects of the global implementation of the technologies in question (Felgner et al., 2018). Whereas highly developed centers use AI, robotics, and intraoperative imaging, most institutes in lower world economies cannot even afford the most basic imaging facility(Menaker et al., 2018). Scalable and cost-effective solutions and the investigation of them in Low-and Middle-Income Countries (LMICs) needs to be done in the future. Such solutions involve the portability of the modular robotic platforms, the affordability of Neuronavigation instruments, and AI diagnostic systems working with the limited cost of computation cloud(Khanna et al., 2021). Also, a cross-border partnership is required to develop open-access surgery datasets and open-source technologies that democratize innovation. Studies are also needed on the existence of alternative approaches to the transfer of technologies, clinical training, and maintenance in underserved locations. The simplified systems can advise policy promotion and funding sources through testing in terms of clinical benefits and cost-efficiency ratio. This digital gap should be narrowed to guarantee equal access to surgery and eliminate the possibility of creating health disparities due to the influence of technology.

8.3 Establishing Ethical and Regulatory Frameworks for Emerging Technologies

In the era of increased data-driven and technology-intensive neurosurgery, the main aim is to formulate strong ethical and regulatory criteria. Future studies will have to cover ethical issues of AI informed clinical decision-making, such as social biases in algorithms, data confidentiality, openness, and legal responsibility in situations involving medical care(Cannizzaro et al., 2022). There have to be guidelines, so as to make sure that machine-generated recommendations are not overriding clinician about the decision-making process or about patient autonomy. Also, the international regulation of advancement like surgical robotics and AI-based diagnosing is still disjointed. The harmonization of international standards of validation, certification, and real-time monitoring of neurosurgical technologies should be studied with research. It is demanded that specific focus is paid to the informed consent in AI-aided procedures as well to make sure that the patients are informed about the work and capacities of these systems(Alves Martins et al., 2023). Moreover, ethical design principles must be incorporated at the development stage of such tools- the focus should be put on the concepts of fairness, accountability, and inclusiveness. By tackling these problems in its own initiative by interdisciplinary research studies, the neurosurgical community will be able to make sure that the further development of the technology will not be opposite to the main ideas of medicine and ethical values of the society.

9. CONCLUSION

The introduction of revolutionary technologies into the cranial and spine surgery process is a game-changer in neurosurgical practice as they combine the power of data-driven intelligence and surgical precision to provide customized, minimally invasive, and results-driven procedures. This chapter has addressed how Artificial Intelligence (AI), Neuronavigation, Intraoperative Imaging, Augmented and Virtual Reality (AR/VR), 3D printing, and robotic-assisted surgery have an immense implication on the entire course of surgery including preoperative planning, the actual surgery and even the postoperative analysis. The case studies of AI-based surgical resection of glioblastoma and robotic spinal fusion have shown that reporting benefits can be transparent and quantitative, such as the precision of the surgical process (up to 98.5%), decreased operative complications, quicker healing and greater patient satisfaction. The given real-life evidence demonstrates that, in case of effective use, transformative tools may provide a decrease in operative time as well as in hospitalization along with the chance of recurrences and, in their turn, improve the level of care in neurosurgery.

Nevertheless, this change does not come without problems. The main obstacles faced on implementing it in large scale include high implementation cost, limited access in low resource setting, lack of training, inconsistency in regulatory frameworks as well as ethical issues on data privacy and algorithmic bias and medico-legal liability. Such obstacles highlight the need to have harmonized strategic plans and interdisciplinary teamwork between neurosurgeons, engineers, data scientists, ethical experts, and policymakers. Another concerning gap in research that the chapter defines is the unavailability of long-term clinical validation research studies and scalable implementation models with many centres, particularly in low and middle-income countries. Regulatory and ethical principles in relation to AI integration, the way to explain algorithmic decision-making to the patients, and the way to obtain informed consent in patients also require further investigation and synchronization. Based on such issues, the chapter recommends the following five pillars: 1) the investment in the long-term training and education, 2) the solution is affordable (through the provision of scalable models of deployment), 3) the protocols and rules should be consistent, 4) all technologies should be ethics-by-design, and 5) cross-disciplinary cooperation should be encouraged. The combination of these measures will be able to reduce the percentage of complications by up to 35-40%, reduce the duration of hospitalization by 30%, and increase the degree of confidence in the AI tools up to 60% The future of neurosurgery is inclusive and collaborative and not merely technological. Closely integrating, continuously reviewing, and committing to fair and patient-centered care is still needed to reach the full potential of the discussed tools and innovations with the great potential they have. The chapter could serve as a reference point in the process of the safe, effective and sustainable implementation of transformative technologies in the neurosurgical practice at the international levels.

ADDITIONAL READING

Chan, E. S. W., Okumus, F., & Chan, W. (2018). Barriers to environmental technology adoption in hotels. *Journal of Hospitality & Tourism Research (Washington, D.C.)*, *42*(5), 829–852.

Parajuli, S., Gyawali, P., Subedi, P., Bhatta, O. P., Mukhia, R., Sedain, G., & Sharma, M. R. (2022). Neurosurgery as a career choice among recent medical graduates from the institute of medicine, Nepal: A cross-sectional study. *Nepal J. Neurosci.*, *19*(4), 39–42.

Yang, V. (2015). Recent advance in visible spectrum surgical navigation. CLEO: 2015.

Zhang, D., Cui, X., Zheng, J., Zhang, S., Wang, M., Lu, W., Sang, L., & Li, W. (2021). Neurosurgical robot-assistant stereoelectroencephalography system: Operability and accuracy. *Brain and Behavior*, *11*(10), e2347. PMID: 34520631

REFERENCES

Alves Martins, B. A., & Filho, O. de M., Ghezzi, T. L., Melani, A. G. F., Romagnolo, L. G. C., Moreira Júnior, H., de Almeida, J. P. P., Araújo, S. E. A., de Sousa, J. B., & de Almeida, R. M. (2023). An overview of robotic colorectal surgsssery adoption and training in Brazil. *Medicina (Kaunas, Lithuania)*, *59*(9). PMID: 37763794

Anyanwu, E. C., Okongwu, C. C., Olorunsogo, T. O., Ayo-Farai, O., Osasona, F., & Daraojimba, O. D. (2024). Artificial Intelligence in healthcare: A review of ethical dilemmas and practical applications. *Imsrj*, *4*(2), 126–140.

Ball, T., González-Mart\'\inez, J., Zemmar, A., Sweid, A., Chandra, S., VanSickle David and Neimat, J. S., Jabbour, P., & Wu, C. (2021). Robotic applications in cranial neurosurgery: Current and future. *Operative Neurosurgery (Hagerstown, Md.)*, *21*(6), 371–379. PMID: 34192764

Benmessaoud, C., Kharrazi, H., & MacDorman, K. F. (2011). Facilitators and barriers to adopting robotic-assisted surgery: Contextualizing the unified theory of acceptance and use of technology. *PLoS One*, *6*(1), e16395. PMID: 21283719

Cannizzaro, D., Zaed, I., Safa, A., Jelmoni, A. J. M., Composto, A., Bisoglio, A., Schmeizer, K., Becker, A. C., Pizzi, A., Cardia, A., & Servadei, F. (2022). Augmented reality in neurosurgery, state of art and future projections. A systematic review. *Frontiers in Surgery*, *9*, 864792. PMID: 35360432

Correa-Arana, K., Vivas-Albán, O. A., & Sabater-Navarro, J. M. (2017). Neurosurgery and brain shift: Review of the state of the art and main contributions of robotics. *TecnoLógicas*, *20*(40), 125–138.

Dennler, C., Bauer, D. E., Scheibler, A.-G., Spirig, J., Götschi, T., Fürnstahl, P., & Farshad, M. (2021). Augmented reality in the operating room: A clinical feasibility study. *BMC Musculoskeletal Disorders*, *22*(1), 451. PMID: 34006234

Felgner, S., Ex, P., & Henschke, C. (2018). Physicians' decision making on adoption of new technologies and role of coverage with evidence development: A qualitative study. *Value in Health*, *21*(9), 1069–1076. PMID: 30224111

Frenkel, C. H. (2023). Telesurgery's evolution during the robotic surgery Renaissance and a systematic review of its ethical considerations. *Surgical Innovation*, *30*(5), 595–600. PMID: 37040578

Hughes-Hallett, A., Mayer, E. K., Marcus, H. J., Cundy, T. P., Pratt, P. J., Parston, G., Vale, J. A., & Darzi, A. W. (2014). Quantifying innovation in surgery. *Annals of Surgery*, *260*(2), 205–211. PMID: 25350647

Hunt, R., Scarpace, L., & Rock, J. (2024). Integration of augmented reality into glioma resection surgery: A case report. *Cureus*, *16*(2), e53573. PMID: 38445166

Javaid, M., Khan, S., Haleem, A., & Rab, S. (2022). Adoption of modern technologies for implementing industry 4.0: An integrated MCDM approach. *Benchmarking*.

Kazemzadeh, K., Akhlaghdoust, M., & Zali, A. (2023a). Advances in artificial intelligence, robotics, augmented and virtual reality in neurosurgery. *Frontiers in Surgery*, *10*, 1241923. PMID: 37693641

Kazemzadeh, K., Akhlaghdoust, M., & Zali, A. (2023b). Advances in artificial intelligence, robotics, augmented and virtual reality in neurosurgery. *Frontiers in Surgery*, *10*, 1241923. PMID: 37693641

Khanna, O., Beasley, R., Franco, D., & DiMaio, S. (2021). The path to surgical robotics in neurosurgery. *Operative Neurosurgery (Hagerstown, Md.)*, *20*(6), 514–520. PMID: 33982116

Konda, N. N., Lewis, T. L., Furness, H. N., Miller, G. W., Metcalfe, A. J., & Ellard, D. R. (2024). Surgeon views regarding the adoption of a novel surgical innovation into clinical practice: Systematic review. *BJS Open*, *8*(1). PMID: 38266120

Konovalov, A., Bykanov, A., Okishev, D., Artemyev, A., Knyazev, A., Ivanov, V., Smirnov, A., Strelkov, S., Pronin, I., Pavlova, G., Pithelauri, D., & Eliava, S. (2024). Augmented Reality Intraoperative Tractography for diffuse glioma microsurgical resection. In *Research Square*.

Lefranc, M., Capel, C., Pruvot, A. S., Fichten, A., & Desenclos, C., Toussaint Patrick and Le Gars, D., & Peltier, J. (2014). The impact of the reference imaging modality, registration method and intraoperative flat-panel computed tomography on the accuracy of the ROSA\textregistered{ } stereotactic robot. *Stereotactic and Functional Neurosurgery*, *92*(4), 242–250. PMID: 25170634

Li, J., Fang, Y., Jin, Z., Wang, Y., & Yu, M. (2020). The impact of robot-assisted spine surgeries on clinical outcomes: A systemic review and meta-analysis. *International Journal of Medical Robotics and Computer Assisted Surgery*, *16*(6), 1–14. PMID: 32725898

Li, W., Li, G., Chen, W., & Cong, L. (2020). The safety and accuracy of robot-assisted pedicle screw internal fixation for spine disease: A meta-analysis. *Bone & Joint Research*, *9*(10), 653–666. PMID: 33101655

Marcus, H. J., Pratt, P., Hughes-Hallett, A., Cundy, T. P., Marcus, A. P., Yang, G.-Z., Darzi, A., & Nandi, D. (2015). Comparative effectiveness and safety of image guidance systems in neurosurgery: A preclinical randomized study. *Journal of Neurosurgery*, *123*(2), 307–313. PMID: 25909567

Mattei, T. A., Rodriguez, A. H., Sambhara, D., & Mendel, E. (2014). Current state-of-the-art and future perspectives of robotic technology in neurosurgery. *Neurosurgical Review*, *37*(3), 357–366. PMID: 24729137

Menaker, S. A., Shah, S. S., Snelling, B. M., Sur, S., Starke, R. M., & Peterson, E. C. (2018). Current applications and future perspectives of robotics in cerebrovascular and endovascular neurosurgery. *Journal of Neurointerventional Surgery*, *10*(1), 78–82. PMID: 28821626

Morimoto, T., & Kobayashi, T., Hirata Hirohito and Otani, K., Sugimoto, M., Tsukamoto, M., Yoshihara, T., Ueno, M., & Mawatari, M. (2022). XR (extended reality: Virtual reality, augmented reality, mixed reality) technology in spine medicine: Status quo and quo Vadis. *Journal of Clinical Medicine*, *11*(2), 470. PMID: 35054164

Olexa, J., Cohen, J., Alexander, T., Brown, C., Schwartzbauer, G., & Woodworth, G. F. (2023). Expanding educational frontiers in neurosurgery: Current and future uses of augmented reality. *Neurosurgery*, *92*(2), 241–250. PMID: 36637263

Pangal, D. J., Cote, D. J., Ruzevick, J., Yarovinsky, B., & Kugener, G., Wrobel Bozena and Ference, E. H., Swanson, M., Hung Andrew J and Donoho, D. A., Giannotta, S., & Zada, G. (2022). Robotic and robot-assisted skull base neurosurgery: Systematic review of current applications and future directions. *Neurosurgical Focus*, *52*(1), E15. PMID: 34973668

Powers, B., Smith, C. D., Arroyo, N., Francis, D. O., & Fernandes-Taylor, S. (2022). How do academic otolaryngologists decide to implement new procedures into practice? *Otolaryngology - Head and Neck Surgery*, *167*(2), 253–261. PMID: 34546818

Robertson, F. C., Wu, K. C., Sha, R. M., Amich, J. M., Lal, A., Lee, B. H., Kirollos, R. W., Chen, M. W., & Gormley, W. B. (2022). Stereotactic neurosurgical robotics with real-time patient tracking: A cadaveric study. *Operative Neurosurgery (Hagerstown, Md.)*, *22*(6), 425–432. PMID: 35867082

Scott, H., Griffin, C., Coggins, W., Elberson, B., Abdeldayem, M., Virmani, T., Larson-Prior, L. J., & Petersen, E. (2021). Virtual reality in the neurosciences: Current practice and future directions. *Frontiers in Surgery*, *8*, 807195. PMID: 35252318

Singh, R., Wang, K., Qureshi, M. B., Rangel, I. C., Brown, N. J., Shahrestani, S., Gottfried, O. N., Patel, N. P., & Bydon, M. (2022). Robotics in neurosurgery: Current prevalence and future directions. *Surgical Neurology International*, *13*(373), 373. PMID: 36128120

Tagaytayan, R., Kelemen, A., & Sik-Lanyi, C. (2018). Augmented reality in neurosurgery. *Archives of Medical Science : AMS, 14*(3), 572–578. PMID: 29765445

Wagner, C. R., Phillips, T., Roux, S., & Corrigan, J. P. (2021). Future directions in robotic neurosurgery. *Operative Neurosurgery (Hagerstown, Md.), 21*(4), 173–180. PMID: 34051701

KEY TERMS AND DEFINITIONS

3D Printing: The process of creating three-dimensional physical models or implants from digital imaging data for pre-surgical planning or patient-specific treatment.

Artificial Intelligence (AI): The capability of machines to simulate human cognitive functions such as learning, reasoning, and decision-making to assist in surgical planning, diagnosis, and real-time interventions.

Augmented Reality (AR): A technology that overlays virtual information such as anatomical structures or surgical plans onto the surgeon's real-world view to improve orientation and visualization.

Ethics-by-Design: An approach that incorporates ethical principles such as fairness, accountability, and privacy into the development and deployment of healthcare technologies.

Explainable AI (XAI): A branch of artificial intelligence designed to make machine-driven decisions interpretable and transparent for human users, particularly clinicians.

Extent of Resection: A clinical measure indicating the proportion (%) of a brain tumor removed during neurosurgery, critical for assessing surgical success and prognosis.

Intraoperative Imaging: Real-time imaging techniques (e.g., MRI, CT, ultrasound) used during surgery to update anatomical views and support accurate decision-making.

Neuronavigation: A computer-assisted technology that guides neurosurgeons during surgery by mapping instruments to preoperative imaging in real time, enhancing precision and safety.

Pedicle Screw Placement: A common spinal fixation technique involving the precise insertion of screws into vertebrae to stabilize the spine, often enhanced by robotic guidance.

Robotic-Assisted Surgery: The use of robotic systems to perform or guide surgical procedures with enhanced control, stability, and precision, especially in minimally invasive spine surgery.

Transformative Neurosurgical Technologies: provides the brief definition of the main terms that are mentioned in the chapter. These terms cut across major technological fields that constitute the emerging core and spine surgeries which are: artificial intelligence, Neuronavigation, robotic and AR/VR. It is critical in order to understand these terms both by clinicians and researchers who are interested in applying or examining these innovations to practice. Such trends as Explainable AI (XAI) or Ethics-by-Design are currently paving the way to the idea of making technology development more open and responsible, especially in the healthcare sector. Meanwhile, Intraoperative Imaging and Extent of Resection are the terms that are directly tied to the outcomes and accuracy of surgical treatment. This glossary can be understood as a ballast to help the readers negotiate the multidisciplinary and complicated language related to neurosurgical transformation.

Chapter 4
AI-Driven Disease Prediction Through Federated Learning:
Privacy-Preserving Innovations in Neurosurgical Technologies

Shaun Liew
Taylor's University, Malaysia

Lim Kean
Taylors University, Malaysia

Soobia Saeed
https://orcid.org/0009-0006-9399-7090
Taylor's University, Malaysia

Lee Seonghyeok
https://orcid.org/0009-0007-0946-3238
Taylor's University, Malaysia

Chong Bitt Shan
Taylors University, Malaysia

Ha XiaoHeng
Taylors University, Malaysia

ABSTRACT

The convergence of artificial intelligence (AI) and neurosurgery has transformed diagnostic precision, preoperative planning, and postoperative monitoring through the integration of advanced data analytics and imaging technologies. However, the centralized storage of sensitive medical data poses significant challenges to patient privacy and data protection, particularly within neurosurgical domains that rely heavily on neuroimaging and electrophysiological datasets. This study explores the implementation of federated learning (FL) as a privacy-preserving approach for AI-driven

DOI: 10.4018/979-8-3373-6234-2.ch004

disease prediction in neurosurgical technologies. The proposed MediPro system integrates convolutional neural networks (CNNs) with federated learning and encrypted communication protocols to analyze MRI and CT scans, offering real-time, AI-assisted preliminary diagnosis while adhering to regulatory standards such as the Personal Data Protection Act (PDPA)

1. INTRODUCTION

In the current world where healthcare has been digitalized so rapidly to the extent that medical data exists in a vast abundance, from electronic health reports to computed tomography (CT) and magnetic resonance imaging (MRI) scans, it is fair to say that it has become much more accessible and efficient to all. However, there are still gaps to plug and improvements to be made, especially in the landscape of healthcare in Malaysia. There exists a significant time lag period in between the time of medical tests and consultations. Patients would often receive the digital copies of their scans or reports as early as the day of the checkup or scan yet are still required to wait days or up to weeks for follow-up physical appointments to receive the diagnosis or know the recommended course of action from a medical professional. This delay may prove to be critical for serious conditions that require early intervention such as cancers or cardiovascular diseases, or just to give a nervous patient peace of mind.

Through the advancement of Artificial Intelligence (AI), machine learning techniques that can learn disease prediction through image analysis and pattern recognition have become quite common. From making use of data mining and AI technology to predict pneumonia cases (Zhang et al., 2024), to being very effective at predicting various types of cancer such as brain, lung, and prostate (B. Zhang et al., 2023), it is clear that AI has come a long way and continues to show potential in the medical industry. However, its implementation still brings challenges in terms of data privacy and security, mainly because of its centralized storing of sensitive patient information. Standard traditional machine learning models require patient data to be collected in a central repository, which still poses a risk under data protection regulations such as the Personal Data Protection Act (PDPA) of Malaysia.

In response to these issues, Federated Learning (FL) is a novel solution that facilitates collaborative training of an AI model across institutions without sharing raw patient data. In neurosurgery, FL supports hospitals and academic institutions to participate in collective AI models, while retaining control of their local neuroimaging datasets to protect patient privacy at their own institutes. This decentralized distributed framework provides advantages not just for data privacy, but for accelerating the development of robust and generalizable predictive models that can assist with complex neurosurgical decision-making, ranging from preoperative risk stratification to postoperative recovery monitoring (Mammen, 2021). This form of learning under decentralized data enhances data privacy and also allows the collaboration of multiple hospitals without fearing data leaks or breaches of sensitive patient information, enhancing the speed and efficiency of building complete AI disease prediction models to be deployed in the medical field. Certain past uses of FL in scenarios such as predicting COVID-19 patients (Dayan et al., 2021) and heart diseases (Kapila & Saleti, 2024) have certainly proven the potential of the integration of federated learning in clinical AI systems. This literature review will go through existing iterations of federated learning integrated into medical systems to observe its feasibility and issues in part of the preparation of a mobile application that leverages federated learning to build a disease prediction model using user- submitted health reports and hospital-generated imaging scans, with the rationale of its design built on bridging the gap of inefficiency in Malaysian healthcare by allowing users to upload reports and scans to receive AI-generated predictions and diagnoses before their next hospital appointment. Through this approach, patients will obtain timely information without delay, improving the efficiency of the healthcare industry.

This research chapter examines the potential for introducing an AI-enabled federated learning to neurosurgical technologies as a method for developing diagnostic systems that are safe, efficient, and intelligent. The research aims to identify gaps in timeliness of diagnosis and security of patient data, specifically with regard to the prediction of disease and in the analysis of neuroimaging data. In discussing the potential of the MediPro framework, this study tries to unlock the promise of federated AI systems to offer predictive advice in real time and to address privacy and ethical obligations. This research establishes a significant opportunity for federated learning to advance privacy-preserving neurosurgical engineering and fundamentally justify the promise of the future of AI-assisted neurosurgery is intelligent but also safe, equitable, and focused on the well-being of the patient.

2.1 Case Studies

2.1.1 Reviewing Federated Machine Learning and Its Use in Diseases Prediction

This review by Moshawrab et al. (2023) explores the usage of Federated Learning (FL) in use cases of disease prediction. Diving into the foundations of FL, the review points out its differences when compared to other machine-learning models and examines how its application fares when used to diagnose diseases such as diabetes, cancer, and cardiovascular conditions.

The decentralized approach to model training is highlighted, as it allows for multiple entities to collaborate and learn from a shared model without the need to exchange raw data. This emphasizes its potential in scenarios where data privacy is important. Such collaborations between institutions help preserve patient privacy as it does not compromise sensitive health data, projecting as a promising approach in the development of AI-driven healthcare solutions going into the future.

Limitations identified include data heterogeneity, as the review notes that varying data distributions across different institutions may pose a challenge to model performance and convergence for FL models. There is also an increased need in communication requirements in FL, which in turn may impact its efficiency, which is especially important in an industry such as the health sector. Lastly, there are still potential vulnerabilities in FL systems that may pose security concerns as FL systems are susceptible to adversarial attacks, hence the need for robust security measures to ensure data breaches do not occur. To potentially address these issues, techniques such as personalized FL or clustering-based FL are suggested to help models adapt to local data in a more effective manner. Model compression and communication-efficient protocols are seen as enhancements for communication efficiency issues, and further exploration of secure aggregation protocols are recommended as ways to mitigate threats such as model inversion or poisoning attacks that may compromise model security.

2.1.2 Review on security of federated learning and its application in healthcare

This review by Li et al. (2023) examines the security challenges faced by FL, specifically within healthcare applications. By diving into various attacks commonly faced such as data and model poisoning and inference attacks, it explores their corresponding defense mechanisms, and through this theme emphasizes the importance of robust security measures in FL systems to protect sensitive patient medical and personal data while still allowing for collaborative model training across different institutions. The defense mechanisms reviewed in the paper include differential privacy, secure multiparty computation, and homomorphic encryption, all of which play a role in mitigating the security threats mentioned above. The emphasis placed on security in this paper further underlines the importance of securing FL systems in healthcare to maintain patient confidentiality and trust.

In terms of limitations, this review notes the absence of standardized datasets and evaluation metrics for assessing the security of FL systems, especially in healthcare. It highlights challenges in balancing data privacy and model performance, as heavier focus being placed on privacy measures can sometimes lower the efficiency of trained models. Lastly, certain defense strategies may not have good scalability with the increasing size and complexity of healthcare data. To improve upon these, suggestions include creating benchmark datasets and metrics tailored to healthcare FL applications that may aid in security assessments; further research into privacy mechanisms that can dynamically provide balance in security as well as model accuracy; and investigating into scalable defense strategies that are capable of handling large scale healthcare data without impacting model performance significantly.

2.1.3 Federated Learning for the Healthcare Metaverse: Concepts, Applications, Challenges, and Future Directions

This Chapter by Bashir et al. (2023) explores the integration of FL within the up-and-coming concept of the Healthcare Metaverse, which is a virtual space enhanced by technologies such as AI, IoT, Augmented or Virtual Reality, and blockchain. With the metaverse holding transformative potential for the healthcare industry through its immersive, personalized, and remote services, there are concerns related to data privacy, security, and interoperability. FL emerges as a promising solution, enabling decentralized model training across multiple institutions without the need to expose sensitive data. A survey on how FL can be used to address these challenges while enabling applications such as disease diagnosis, remote patient monitoring, medical education, and pandemic management is carried out in this paper.

Distinguishing between conventional healthcare systems and healthcare in the Metaverse, the ability of immersive technologies to potentially improve training, diagnosis and treatments is highlighted, as well as the benefits of FL being used in such a system, providing better privacy, data management, automation, and scalability. It also proposes a layered architecture of the Healthcare Metaverse, including infrastructure, human interfaces, decentralization, spatial computing, and more. Emphasis is also placed on the ability FL has to mitigate issues such as data bias and privacy, while still maintaining the stance that real-time decision making should still be a necessity in the Metaverse.

However, the paper still remains largely theoretical, and there is a need for empirical evaluation of FL models in a live healthcare Metaverse environment. Detailed strategies on privacy preservation are not analyzed on a deeper level in the paper, and the effectiveness of deploying FL on resource-constrained devices in high-latency environments remain to be seen. Regulatory compliances in cross-border data processing within the Metaverse is also not addressed clearly. Even so, the paper lays a solid foundation on the application of FL models in the healthcare sector.

2.1.4 Federated Learning for Neurosurgical Applications: A Taxonomy, Current Trends, Challenges, and Future Research Directions

Rauniyar et al. (2023) conducted a study which not only presents a thorough classification but also critical evaluation of FL frameworks used in the medical sector, pointing out their function in the development of privacy-preserving AI. In the case of neurosurgery, FL is an entirely new way of dealing with sensitive neuroimaging and patient data; these can be used for diagnosis and predicting outcomes even without disclosing the patient's identity. The whole model training process is distributed among various neurosurgery centers, and research institutions; thus, there is no need to share any raw data at all, and so the very strict data protection regulations like the

Personal Data Protection Act (PDPA) and HIPAA are fully complied with. This is very important since the management of highly sensitive neurological patient records relies heavily on these regulations. Rauniyar and others (2023) have divided federated learning (FL) into three types: horizontal, vertical and federated transfer learning models, with each model being suitable for a specific neurosurgical data environment. Among hospitals with similar imaging modalities, such as MRI or CT scans of brain tumors, horizontal FL enables collaboration, whereas vertical FL facilitates integration across the institutions with data types that are complementary, such as combining neuroimaging with electrophysiological or genomic datasets. Federated transfer learning offers further flexibility as it allows the local datasets to refine the pre-trained neurosurgical AI models for the optimization specific to that site. The combination of FL with new technologies—like blockchain for secure data exchange, IoT-based neuromonitoring systems, and edge computing for intraoperative AI support— was not only beneficial for data privacy but also made the neurosurgical environment more scalable.

In neurosurgery, where AI-enhanced federated models can help with early tumor categorization, surgical planning, and postoperative outcome prediction, the chapter's mentioned applications—such as disease prediction for brain tumors and cancers—are especially pertinent. Decentralized neurosurgical AI systems that can collaborate in real time between research labs and academic hospitals can be developed using open-source frameworks like FedML and TensorFlow Federated. Even with these developments, a number of significant obstacles still exist. Model generalization may be hampered statistically by the non-independent and non-identically distributed (non-IID) character of neuroimaging data across institutions. Large-scale implementation is also hampered by system-related problems, such as erratic internet access or client outages during model synchronization. From a security standpoint, the accuracy of AI-assisted neurosurgical diagnosis is seriously threatened by adversarial assaults and model poisoning.

The paper concludes by highlighting the lack of benchmarking measures and standardized neurosurgical datasets for assessing FL systems, which restrict their transfer from research prototypes to clinical use. To prove FL-based neurosurgical instruments' clinical viability and regulatory compliance, extensive, multi-institution validation studies are required. In order to guarantee that AI-driven advancements continue to improve surgical accuracy and patient safety while maintaining data integrity and privacy, future research should concentrate on creating scalable, interpretable, and clinically proven FL architectures specifically designed for neurosurgical imaging.

2.1.5 Federated Learning and Homomorphic Encryption for Secure Neurosurgical Diagnostics

To protect sensitive medical data during online diagnosis, Shen et al. (2023) presented a safe and effective federated learning (FL) architecture that incorporates homomorphic encryption. By employing blinded local parameters to ensure absolute secrecy, the model allows several hospitals to work together to build a global diagnostic algorithm without exchanging raw patient data. The Okamoto–Uchiyama (OU) cryptosystem and a Support Vector Machine (SVM) classifier are used in the system to provide encrypted computation and real-time disease prediction with low communication costs.

A system like this has great potential for safely evaluating MRI and CT neuroimaging data from a neurosurgical standpoint, enabling AI-assisted predictions for diseases like brain tumors, intracranial bleeding, and neurodegenerative disorders while protecting patient privacy. On real-world datasets, the method showed high diagnosis accuracy (85.9–98.6%), demonstrating its effectiveness and scalability for clinical usage across multiple institutions. The study did point out some drawbacks, though, most notably the lack of differential privacy safeguards, the dependence on an offline, reliable third party to distribute encryption keys, and the constraint to binary classification models, which may hinder sophisticated neurosurgical applications. In order to better capture complex neuroanatomical patterns and improve predictive accuracy while upholding strict data privacy norms, future research should investigate incorporating deep neural networks within secured FL systems.

3. METHODOLOGY

3.1 System Analysis

The purpose of the system analysis is to identify and articulate the needed technical, functional, and non-functional requirements of a federated-learning AI-based system aimed at predicting neurosurgical diseases and providing decision support. The study is focused on establishing an approach that integrates decentralized learning models, improving diagnostic accuracy, protecting patient care data privacy, and optimizing clinician workflow within the field of neurosurgery.

The proposed system, MediPro Neuro, intends to address problems currently encountered in the neurosurgical diagnostic process and, more specifically, the time difference between diagnostic imaging (CT, MRI) and clinical appointments. Often, patients receive their imaging results in a timely manner, however they may then have to wait days and weeks for a specialist to review those images and plan for surgical intervention. This lag is particularly harmful in acute neurological disorders, including brain tumors, intracranial hemorrhages, and spinal cord compression, where timely diagnosis and surgical treatment matters.

With federated learning (FL), the system allows multiple neurosurgery centers and hospitals to collectively train AI models utilizing distributed clinical neuroimaging data while keeping sensitive patient health information decentralized. This helps adhere to privacy legislation, such as the Personal Data Protection Act (PDPA) and HIPAA, while also increasing the model's diversity and generalizability. The AI component, utilizing convolutional neural networks (CNNs), analyzes MRI and CT scans to identify pathologies including gliomas, meningiomas, and TBI, offering predictive insights into clinical decision-making in real time for the neurosurgeons.

The stakeholder-centered design framework is part of the system analysis. The stakeholders are neurosurgeons, radiologists, hospital IT administrators, patients, and AI developers. Each is critical to delivering a solution that is clinically relevant, technically secure, and ethically sound. Neurosurgeons and radiologists provide domain expertise in the labeling and validating of diagnostic imaging. From the perspective of engineers working on the AI model, technicians focus on model architecture and securing data from patients. Patients benefit by receiving a predictive assessment early with less latency in receiving a surgical diagnosis, allowing patients to be better prepared and have better mental well-being prior to their surgical consultation.

In summary, the MediPro Neuro system is designed to implement a secure, user-friendly, and scalable digital solution for neurosurgical care. The project is an attempt to incorporate federated learning and neuroimaging advanced analytical techniques to bridge the potential gap between acquiring imaging studies and surgical decision making, while providing increased precision and privacy in the context of the distinctiveness of current practice in neurosurgery.

3.2 Stakeholder Analysis

To succeed in building an application that checks all the marks, understanding the involved stakeholders plays an important role.

3.2.1 Patients/Users

Patients represent the key end users of this application and who it is tailored to. Through the application, users can upload soft copies of their health reports or CT/MRI scans obtained from the hospital they have visited, to then receive an AI prediction along with generated reports or recommendations on further courses of action. Users should be expecting ease of usage of the application, clarity, data privacy, and timely feedback.

3.2.2 Developers

Developers are the stakeholders in charge of the overall design of the application, as well as maintaining the federate learning models, database and machine learning algorithms. Their emphasis will be on ensuring model accuracy, scalability and data security.

3.2.3 Hospitals and Medical Institutions

The stakeholders in charge of actually providing important medical information via their patient scans or body checks. The imaging data from scans and e-health reports provided by hospitals and medical institutions will be contributed to the federated learning models and algorithms. At the same time, hospitals and medical institutions will be allowed access to the prediction models themselves if needed.

3.2.4 Investors

Investors in the application will be interested in understanding its technical feasibility and its potential on the market, looking for cost-effectiveness and its overall utility provided.

Figure 1. Use Case Diagram

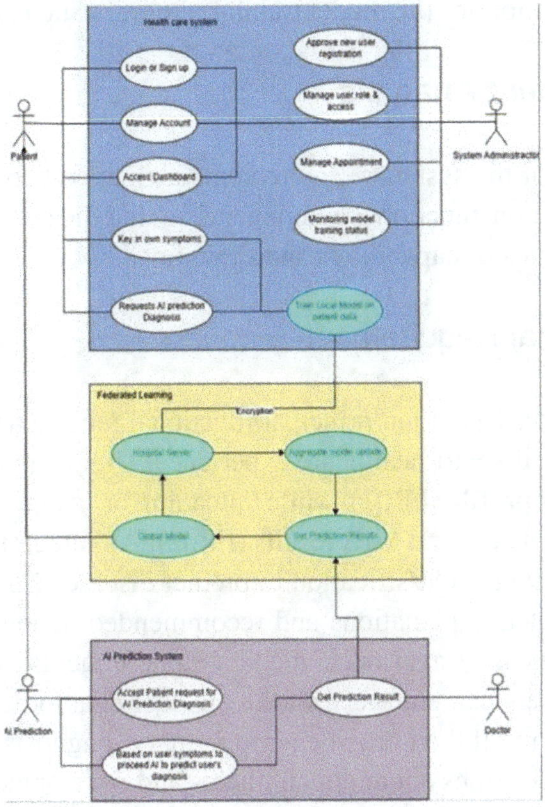

The diagram above shows the use case diagram of the MediPro application, showing the functions available to the users and system admins, as well as a look into the federated learning system and AI prediction system. As shown above, patients or otherwise the users will be able to login or sign up for the system, manage their account and access the dashboard. Through "keying in their own symptoms" or otherwise uploading the soft copies of their CT and MRI scans or health reports, they can request for AI predictions from the system. Through the federated learning system, this data from the local server is then trained. As shown in the federated learning segment, data from hospital servers will be used to aggregate the model update. The prediction results will then be obtained and are sent to the global model, which is lastly sent back to the local hospital server. Doctors will also have access to view prediction results and validate them straight from the AI prediction model itself. As for system admins, they will have access to approve of new user registrations, manage user role and access, manage appointments made by users, as well as monitor the model training progress and status.

3.3 Requirement Analysis

The analysis of the system's requirements is divided between functional components and non-functional components so that the system can be fully understood in terms of capabilities and limitations.

3.3.1 Functional Requirement

The system consists of ten principal functional requirements for providing a seamless and smart healthcare experience. Users can register, log in, and manage their profile (FR01), while uploading or scanning their medical documents, such as CT and MRI results (FR02). An integrated CNN-based model performs image classification to predict diseases (FR03) while also providing annotated explanations and recommended actions generated by AI (FR04). Users may also book medical appointments within the platform (FR05). Users can engage with the eDoctor chatbot to describe their symptoms, which will then provide a preliminary diagnosis (FR06). Users will receive notifications about appointments and developments in a timely manner (FR07), export their results to pdf (FR08), and will have access to a complete history log of previous scans with predicted outcomes (FR09). Finally, the results will be displayed through a clear visualization interface that creates an engaging user experience (FR10).

3.3.2 Non-Functional Requirements

The non-functional requirements for the system include reliability, security, and scalability for the intended use of the system. Performance will need to run quickly and efficiently, with the full scan analysis being completed within 20 seconds (NFR01). To secure user data, the system should encrypt user data and comply with the Personal Data Protection Act (PDPA) (NFR02). Usability will be emphasized with a simplistic, guided user interface (NFR03). The system will also have scalability considerations, supporting up to 20,000 active users, as well as accommodating efficient performance for more data volume (NFR04). To ensure continuous access, high availability service considerations should be included, targeting 99% uptime (NFR05). Maintainability will also be a requirement, allowing for easy updates and fixes be implemented into the system (NFR06). Interoperability of any medical data will also be included (DICOM and PDF) (NFR07). The system will need to support both structured and unstructured data to support the intended analysis (NFR08). The AI prediction model will also need to be accurate, maintaining at least a 97% diagnostic accuracy, and will be retrained regularly as appropriate (NFR09). It will also be critical that any APIs are integrated and have latency time attempts, regardless of large-scale integrated response time (NFR10).

3.4 Feasibility Study

3.4.1 SWOT Analysis

Strong privacy safeguards, interpretability of results, AI-driven diagnostic prediction capabilities, and the system's capacity to close the gap between clinical consultations and diagnostic imaging are some of its advantages. Nevertheless, it has drawbacks like high processing requirements, reliance on other APIs, possible problems with user trust, and reliance on the caliber of data submitted. The growing digital healthcare market in Malaysia, probable development into other medical specialties, and potential cooperation with governmental or non-governmental initiatives represent important opportunities. On the other hand, risks include cybersecurity flaws, ethical dilemmas including model bias, competition from comparable healthcare apps, and strict regulatory restrictions.

3.5 Risk Analysis

3.5.1 Data Privacy

MediPro will have to deal with sensitive information about hospital patients, which means a risk of data breaches will always be present, and thus will need strong encryption protocols as well as regulatory compliance such as the PDPA. More specifically, federated learning will help with this problem by reducing the need for raw data sharing.

3.5.2 AI Prediction Accuracy

When AI predictions are incorrect and/or inaccurate, it could negatively impact users' trust, particularly when very negative predictions are provided. This is why models should be maintained and retrained on a regular basis and disclaimers should suggest that they seek professional medical advice favorably.

3.5.3 User Usability

Encouraging users of all ages to utilize the application requires a user experience that is responsive, easy to grasp, and intuitive. User testing of prototypes is crucial to accomplishing this in order to comprehend and get input for future development.

3.5.4 Scalability and System Performance

The application must continue to operate consistently and optimally given the volume of medical data and information gathered. For scalability, the back-end frameworks and architecture must be properly connected with cloud-based storage.

3.6 Data Types and Models

3.6.1 Medical Imaging Data (CT/MRI Scans)

CT and MRI scans are high-resolution medical images, providing detailed anatomical information used for the diagnosing of diseases. They are typically stored in DICOM or PDF formats, which are then converted into image data to be used for analysis purposes. These data are often complex and multi-dimensional, requiring well-built deep learning models that are capable of extracting features such as various textures and patterns and detect anomalies from images of tissue, organ structures and so on.

3.6.2 Convolutional Neural Network (CNN) for Image Classification

Well-known for its image classification capabilities, CNN will be used as the core structure of MediPro's image analysis component thanks to its ability to detect spatial structures which are useful for image data (Guo & Zhu, 2019). The CNN model will be trained on CT and MRI datasets obtained from medical institutions for the identification of disease-related patterns such as various types of tumors, lumps, or anomalies in human organs. In addition, these CNN models are trained in a federated learning manner across different hospital and medical institution datasets, ensuring vast varieties and patient data privacy.

3.6.3 Text-based Health Reports

Digital health reports, which include lab results and clinical notes, are often presented as semi- structured or unstructured data that contain vital patient information such as anomalies and symptoms, blood pressure levels, blood sugar levels, and so on. Such data, when presented alongside data from imaging scans, can provide good context for AI predictions and assist the AI when generating recommendations and explanations in layman terms understandable to the general public.

3.6.4 Third-Party APIs for Explanations and Recommendations

To provide easily understandable explanations, the MediPro system will integrate third-party APIs such as those of ChatGPT or DeepSeek. These models will be used to generate summaries in layman terms understandable by users regarding the results of their imaging scan data or health reports. They will also provide health recommendations or questions that can be then asked during an actual consultation with medical professionals. Its goal is not to directly replace medical professionals and practitioners, but to be a helpful assistant to them aiding patients better understand their own health and conditions.

4. SYSTEM DESIGN

This chapter will go through the system design for MediPro, a federated learning-based AI disease prediction application. A system architecture diagram showing the integration of its various components will be included, along with a storyboard of scenarios of user interaction with the application as well as the features in the prototype of the user interface.

Figure 2. System Architecture Diagram

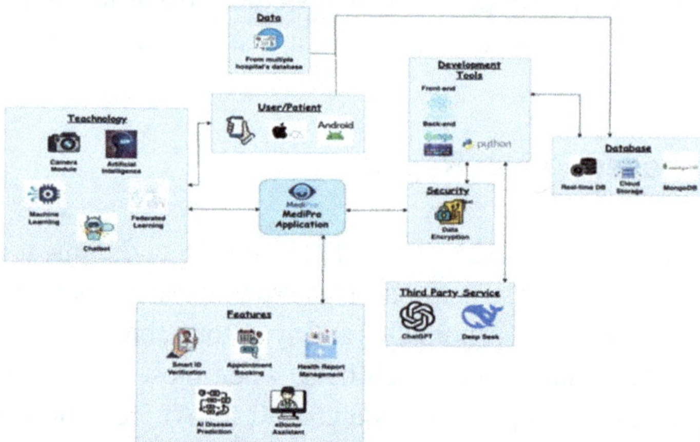

Figure 2 Shown above is the system architecture diagram of each component in the system of the MediPro application. With data encryption and the federated learning system part of the security layer, the application will be developed using React on the front-end for its component-based UI development and Django on the back end for its rapid development process through the use of Python. Third-party API services such as ChatGPT and DeepSeek will be integrated for easily interpreted recommendation and explanation generation. Data obtained via hospital or medical institution servers such as CT/MRI scans and e-health reports will be stored in real-time cloud storage based databases through the integration of MongoDB. End users, or in this case patients, will be able to access the application through their mobile phones, accessing its features provided including smart ID verification, appointment booking, health report management, AI disease prediction, eDoctor assistant and so on. These features are made possible through technology used in the application such as the camera module to scan images, AI and chatbots to

generate recommendations, machine learning to train disease prediction models, and federated learning for the privacy aspect of the research work.

4.1 User Interface Design

4.1.1 Welcome Page

Upon entering the application, users will be greeted by the welcome page, consisting of the MediPro logo. Text welcoming the user will appear, along with a prompt to select the current medical institution the user is visiting. Upon confirmation, a loading screen will appear to indicate the system is starting up as shown in Figure 3.

Figure 3. Login page of MediPro

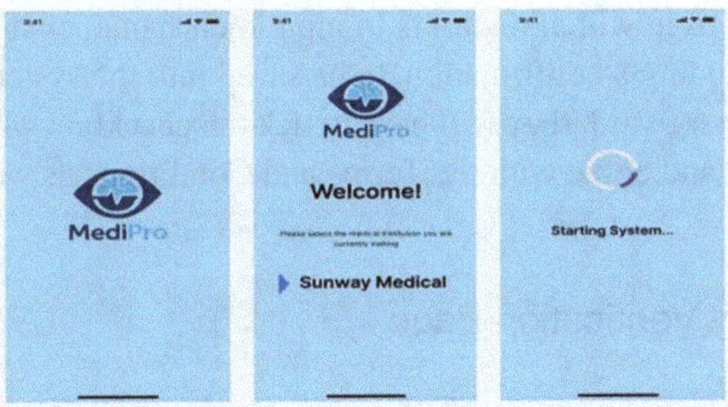

4.1.2 Login/Signup Page

A login page with multiple options of logging in will appear for the user, requiring their email address and associated password. Alternatively, users can continue on through Google, Apple ID or Facebook. If they have yet to register, they can do so via a prompt underneath the Login button that says, "Register now". In cases of a wrong email or password, the screen on the right will appear to alert users of a wrong email or password as shown in Figure 4.

Figure 4. Welcome page

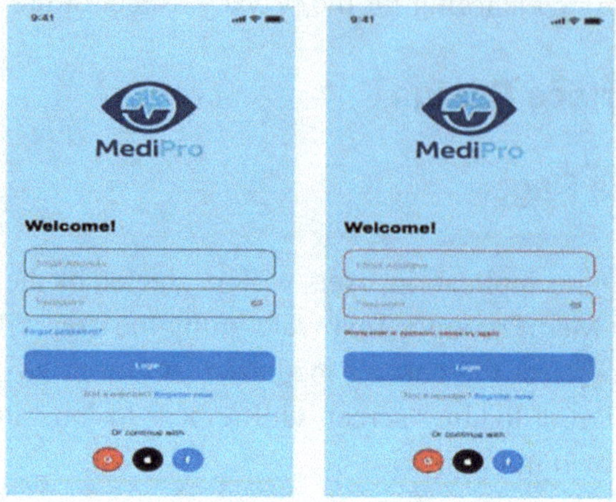

The signup page will allow users to input their name, email address and password, including a confirmation, to be saved into the system's database. Before moving forward, they will have to tick the checkbox which confirms they have read and agree with the Terms and Conditions as well as Privacy Policy.

4.1.3 Identity Verification Page

For identity verification, users are required to go through two steps of verification, being the document verification step and the facial verification step. The document verification page requires users to scan the front side of their identification card to continue, before prompting a facial verification step in which users will have to scan their face in the frame provided as shown in Figure 5.

Figure 5. User identification

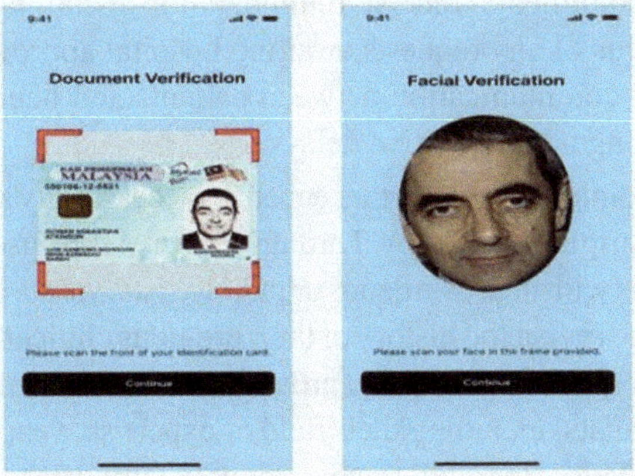

4.1.4 User Interface Components

The dashboard serves as the central interface of the MediPro Neuro application, offering users an intuitive overview of all available features. At the top of the screen, the user's name and profile image are displayed, alongside a notification icon for quick access to alerts and updates. Directly below, a prominent "Make Appointment" button allows users to schedule consultations seamlessly. The central portion of the dashboard contains interactive buttons for the application's primary neurosurgical functions, including "Health Report Diagnosis," "eDoctor," and "AI Prediction." Each of these features enables users to upload or review their CT and MRI neuroimaging scans, receive AI-generated diagnostic insights, and access professional guidance through the integrated virtual assistant. The bottom section of the dashboard provides personalized educational materials, such as videos and articles curated by an algorithm that tailors content based on the user's medical history and past AI prediction results. For instance, a patient whose MRI analysis reveals indications of a brain tumor may be presented with neurosurgeon-recommended rehabilitation guides or informative videos about preoperative preparation. At the very top, a dropdown menu allows users to select or update the medical institution currently overseeing their scans, ensuring that the system retrieves and processes the correct data for prediction and follow-up purposes.

The notifications page functions as the user's centralized alert center, providing real-time updates regarding their neurosurgical appointments, diagnostic reports, and AI analysis results. Here, users can review confirmed and pending appointments, receive reminders for upcoming consultations, and track the status of any requests awaiting hospital approval. This feature ensures efficient communication between patients and neurosurgical institutions, minimizing administrative delays.

The make appointment page further enhances accessibility and coordination within the neurosurgical workflow. Through this interface, users can schedule new consultations with neurosurgeons or radiologists, view a list of upcoming appointments, and revisit the history of their previous clinical visits. The page also allows for easy rescheduling and provides detailed information about the consulting specialists, including their field of expertise, years of experience, and availability. This integrated system not only simplifies patient–hospital interaction but also ensures timely access to professional neurosurgical care, bridging the gap between AI-based disease prediction and clinical follow-up as shown in Figure 6.

Figure 6. Select Specialization page

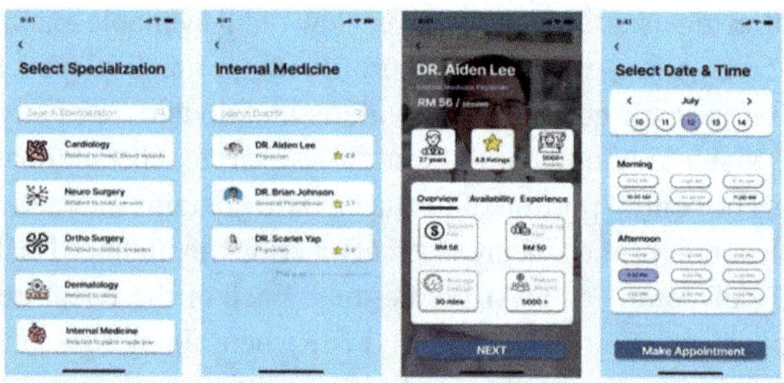

Figure 7. Appointment page

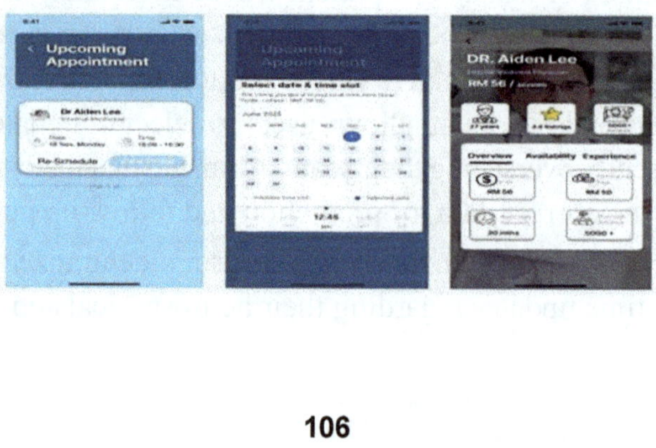

Upcoming appointments allow users to check any upcoming appointments they made, along with an option to reschedule them or check on the doctor's profile as shown in Figure 7.

Figure 8. Past Appointment Page

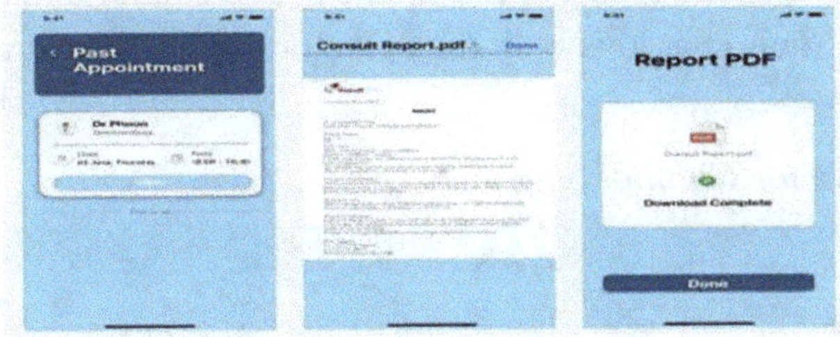

Past appointment page allows users to check history of their past appointments and download the consultation report in PDF format. Health Report Diagnosis Page allows a user to scan their physical health reports, also allowing for the option to retake the photo as shown in Figure 8.

Figure 9. Upload report page

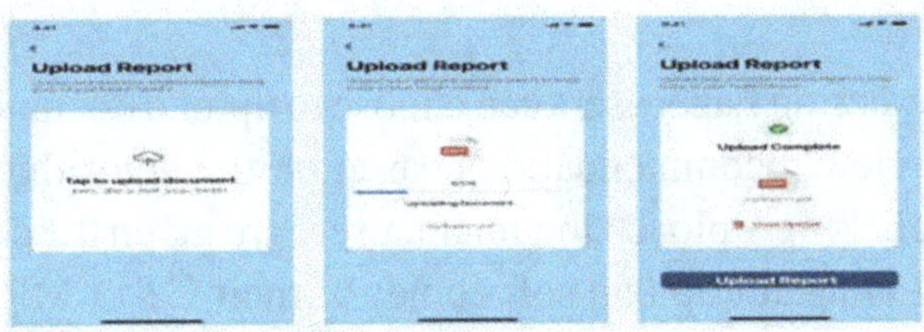

Alternatively, users can upload PDF copies of their health reports. Users can then save the details and information of the health report in the database of the system, being able to write a name for the report, its type, and date. Users can have an AI Diagnosis generated based on their health reports, obtaining an explanation of each statistic and condition in layman terms as well as generating recommended course of actions as shown in Figure 9.

4.1.5 eDoctor Chatbot Page

Through the eDoctor Chatbot page, users can interact with a chatbot assistant and tell it their symptoms or condition, in which the eDoctor will generate a diagnosis after analyzing it and provide a clear message of recommendations. Users can then save the reports generated by the eDoctor and also view the past history of their chat logs with the eDoctor as shown in Figure 10.

Figure 10. eDoctor Chatbot page

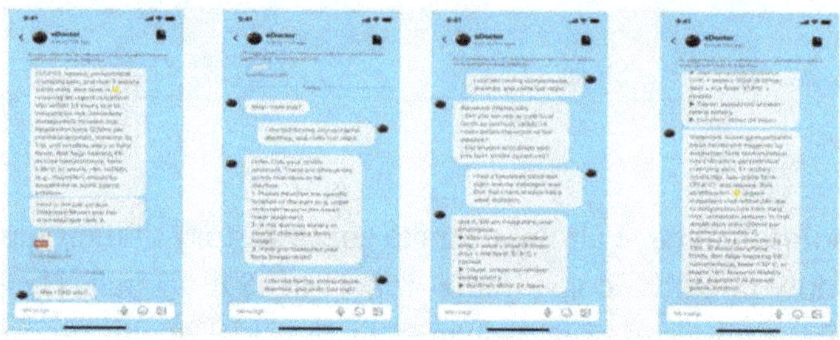

4.1.6 AI Disease Prediction Page

In the AI Prediction Page, users can choose to upload documents, generate AI report, and view recommendations based on the algorithm of their past records. After clicking Upload Document, users are given the choice to either scan a physical image or upload soft copies of their CT or MRI scans. They can also view the history of their previous images as shown in Figure 11.

Figure 11. CT/PET Scan details page

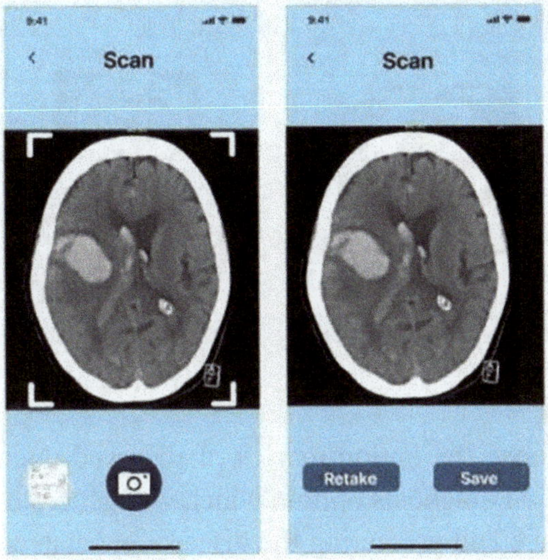

Users can either choose to scan a physical image, or upload PDF or documents of their scans.

Figure 12. Documents page

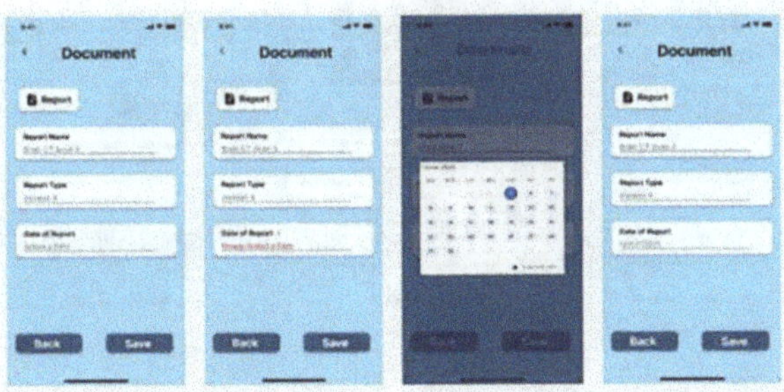

Users will then be able to save their scanned documents, filling in report name, report type, and its date as shown in Figure 12.

Figure 13. AI prediction page

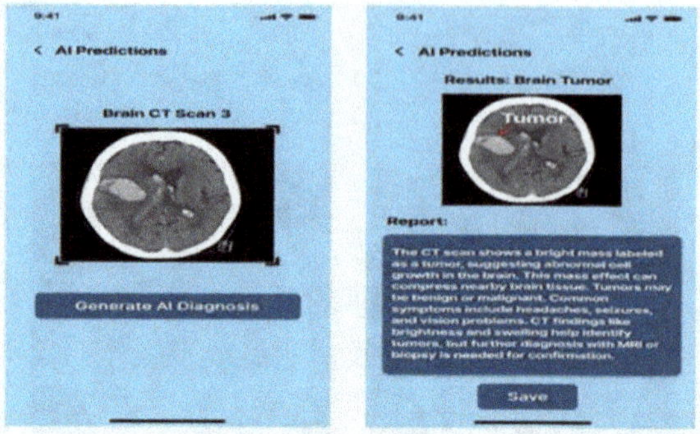

After users choose the option to view their saved documents, they can click the generate AI diagnosis option, which will generate a diagnosis after analyzing the image and predicting the disease associated with it as shown in Figure 13.

Figure 14. AI prediction Reports

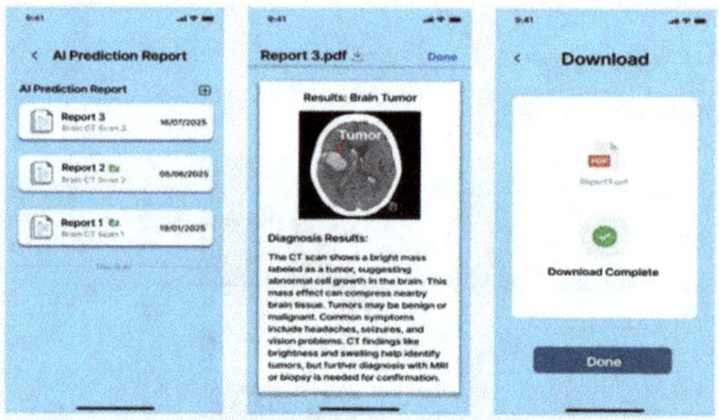

Users can then save the AI prediction reports, view them again, or download them for use in consultations with doctors as shown in Figure 14.

5. DISCUSSION

The application of artificial intelligence (AI) and federated learning (FL) to neurosurgical technologies is shifting the paradigm for diagnostic and decision support systems. The results from the literature indicated that FL provides a realistic and ethically responsible method for the safe use of distributed neurosurgical data, especially in the case of sensitive neuroimaging data from modalities like MRI and CT. Traditional centralized AI systems compromise patients' privacy by conglomerating data into a centralized repository, creating risks related to the data protection regulations in place such as the Personal Data Protection Act (PDPA) in Malaysia and HIPAA. In contrast, FL permits hospitals and neurosurgical centers to train AI without sharing patient data outside the clinician's institution, maintaining confidentiality while improving model reliability.

In neurosurgery, rapid identification and accurate interpretation of images are important determinants of surgical outcomes. FL's decentralized approach supports developing collaborative models that can leverage data from different institutions, a feature that improves the generalizability of AI-based predictions in conditions such as brain tumors, intracranial hemorrhage, spinal cord injury, and related conditions. Rauniyar et al. (2023) and Shen et al. (2023) demonstrated improvement in model security and diagnostic efficiency through data aggregation combined with FL and encryption, such as homomorphic encryption, spanning accuracy levels of 85.9%-98.6%. Such hybrid models are particularly useful in neurosurgical contexts due to the high dimensionality of image data that requires both the accuracy and computation of AI, with monitoring of encrypted data.

Although some difficulties still exist in utilizing FL in neurosurgical settings. One of the issues that that the imaging centers generate different data quality, and this won't help since the model will have different convergences and different stable predictions. In addition, large neuroimaging datasets would impose heavy computational and communication overheads that will possibly make training slower, especially in hospitals with limited resources. There are still security threats like model poisoning, adversarial attacks and potential inference leaks which are some of the risks that need to be addressed using differential privacy and secure aggregation methods. It is also necessary that there is a universal standard for neurosurgical datasets and metrics for benchmarking so that the evaluation of FL frameworks can be carried out uniformly across different hospitals.

The MediPro Neuro system, which was developed in this research, tackles several of these problems by the use of a federated convolutional neural network (CNN) architecture specifically tailored for neurosurgical disease prediction. Its design merges secure encryption layers, cloud-based data synchronization, and third-party APIs for interpretability and patient communication. This all-embracing method connects the two worlds of imaging diagnostics and surgical consultations by giving patients early predictive insights and equipping neurosurgeons with AI-assisted interpretation tools. The MediPro Neuro system achieves a major reduction in diagnostic latency, which makes it easier to move towards the future of a more proactive, data-secure, and patient-centered model of neurosurgical care.

6. CONCLUSION

The integration of federated learning into neuro-surgical related technologies opens up a revolutionary avenue to improve diagnostic accuracy, ensure patient privacy and better utilize clinical workflows. This research highlights how decentralized Artificial Intelligence (AI) applied within the MediPro Neuro framework can solve existing challenges encountered while collecting and analyzing large neuro-surgical databases. Rather than sharing neuroimaging datasets, medical institutions can collaborate to train AI models in a decentralized network, allowing for data privacy compliance while producing improved diagnostic accuracy, clinical applicability and generalizability.

The combination of federated convolutional neural networks (CNNs), secure encryption protocols, and explainable AI user interfaces represent an essential evolution in building more ethical and intelligent neurosurgical systems. Ongoing challenges exist in the fields of neurosurgical practice including data heterogeneity, energy cost of the models and lack of standardized methodologies for research to collaborate operationally, but as neuro-surgical fields continue to improve methods of coding and multiple hospitals collaborate with other sites to test FL and models, the credibility of federated learning's clinical applicability will improve.

In conclusion, while there remain challenges to utilizing AI-assisted neurosurgery, to ensure that diagnostic outcomes are safer, faster and more individualized, the potential exists to shape the future of AI-assisted neurosurgery. As health care systems drift toward precision medicine, privacy-preserving technologies, such as FL, bridge data-driven precision into evidence-based practices and assure that education and practice in neurosurgery and health care remain connected to ethical practices.

REFERENCES

Bashir, A. K., Victor, N., Bhattacharya, S., Huynh-The, T., Chengoden, R., Yenduri, G., & Liyanage, M. (2023). Federated learning for the healthcare metaverse: Concepts, applications, challenges, and future directions. *IEEE Internet of Things Journal, 10*(24), 21873–21891.

Dayan, I., Roth, H. R., Zhong, A., Harouni, A., Gentili, A., Abidin, A. Z., Liu, A., Costa, A. B., Wood, B. J., Tsai, C., Wang, C., Hsu, C., Lee, C. K., Ruan, P., Xu, D., Wu, D., Huang, E., Kitamura, F. C., Lacey, G., & Li, Q. (2021). Federated learning for predicting clinical outcomes in patients with COVID-19. *Nature Medicine, 27*(10), 1735–1743. DOI: 10.1038/s41591-021-01506-3 PMID: 34526699

Guo, A. J. X., & Zhu, F. (2019). A CNN-based spatial feature fusion algorithm for hyperspectral imagery classification. *IEEE Transactions on Geoscience and Remote Sensing, 57*(9), 7170–7181. DOI: 10.1109/TGRS.2019.2911993

Kapila, R., & Saleti, S. (2024). Federated learning-based disease prediction: A fusion approach with feature selection and extraction. *Biomedical Signal Processing and Control, 100*, 106961. DOI: 10.1016/j.bspc.2024.106961

Li, H., Li, C., Wang, J., Yang, A., Ma, Z., Zhang, Z., & Hua, D. (2023). Review on security of federated learning and its application in healthcare. *Future Generation Computer Systems, 144*, 271–290. DOI: 10.1016/j.future.2023.02.021

Mammen, P. M. (2021, January 14). *Federated learning: Opportunities and challenges.* arXiv.org. https://arxiv.org/abs/2101.05428

Moshawrab, M., Adda, M., Bouzouane, A., Ibrahim, H., & Raad, A. (2023). Reviewing federated machine learning and its use in diseases prediction. *Sensors (Basel), 23*(4), 2112. DOI: 10.3390/s23042112 PMID: 36850717

Rauniyar, A., Hagos, D. H., Jha, D., Håkegård, J. E., Bagci, U., Rawat, D. B., & Vlassov, V. (2023). Federated learning for medical applications: A taxonomy, current trends, challenges, and future research directions. *IEEE Internet of Things Journal, 11*(5), 7374–7398.

Shen, G., Fu, Z., Gui, Y., Susilo, W., & Zhang, M. (2023). Efficient and privacy-preserving online diagnosis scheme based on federated learning in e-healthcare system. *Information Sciences*, *647*, 119261. DOI: 10.1016/j.ins.2023.119261

Zhang, B., Shi, H., & Wang, H. (2023). Machine learning and AI in cancer prognosis, prediction, and treatment selection: A critical approach. *Journal of Multidisciplinary Healthcare*, *16*, 1779–1791. DOI: 10.2147/JMDH.S410301 PMID: 37398894

Zhang, J., Yang, P., Zeng, L., Li, S., & Zhou, J. (2024). Ventilator-associated pneumonia prediction models based on AI: Scoping review. *JMIR Medical Informatics*, *12*, e57026. DOI: 10.2196/57026 PMID: 38771220

Chapter 5
Implementation of Neuronavigation-Guided Resection in Complex Intracranial Tumors

Rubina Ghani
https://orcid.org/0000-0003-1923-7924
Sohail University, Pakistan

ABSTRACT

The chapter presents cutting-edge surgical advances, neuronavigation, intraoperative MRI (iMRI), and 5-aminolevulinic acid (5-ALA) fluorescence-guided resection techniques for treating complex intracranial tumors and their implications for clinical care. These advances allow the surgeon to visualize the tumor in real time and know where the tumor begins and ends—all of which improve surgical accuracy, decrease complications and increase extents of resection (EOR). Neuronavigation, often described as a "GPS for the brain," uses data from multiple imaging modalities (CT, MRI, and functional studies) to develop an intraoperative 3D map of the intraoperative anatomy. This increases surgical finesse, reduces the injury to normal brain, and promotes more aggressive tumor resection. The development of neuronavigation has changed from the initial stereotactic frame, to incorporating a frameless intraoperative mapping approach to now being image-integrated (providing dynamic image updates)—and provides an important opportunity to improve surgical precision.

DOI: 10.4018/979-8-3373-6234-2.ch005

1. INTRODUCTION

Neurosurgeons can bring images of the patient's brain into the operating room to improve surgical approaches. At some point, any digital scan—CT, MRI or PET—can be loaded onto a workstation in the operating room. When necessary, multiple image sets can be joined together through a process called registration. With the help of specially placed skin markers or the patient's own anatomy, the image information can now be referenced to the patient. This provides information to the surgeon, allowing them to touch any point in the surgical field and see it appear on the workstation screen. With this information, the exact contours of a tumor can be mapped prior to surgery (Malbert, 2021).

Clinically, the identification of central nervous system (CNS) lesions became impractical in the 19th and 20th centuries, as clinicians developed an understanding of the spatial organization of functional areas in the nervous system. Anatomical and functional localization progressed alongside the advent of imaging tools such as angiography and air ventriculography, and subsequently, various cross-sectional imaging techniques (e.g., computed tomography (CT) and magnetic resonance imaging (MRI)). To more accurately place tumors and nonneoplastic surgical targets, we developed the stereotactic coordinate system and headframe. As frameless navigational systems developed, studies showed that the logistical issues of frame-based stereotactic navigations could be minimized (Sulangi et.al, 2025).

In the future, as the ability to perform multimodal neuronavigation is incorporated into commercially available clinical systems, surgeons will have more and more options to help them biopsy and resect brain tumors.

1.1 Overview of Gliomas

Glioma represents the most common type of tumor within the central nervous system, originating from glial cells. It is distinguished by its diffuse infiltration of adjacent brain tissue; among gliomas, glioblastoma is recognized as the most aggressive variant, while pilocytic astrocytoma is regarded as the least malignant (Ostrom et al., 2023).

According to information from the CBTRUS, gliomas represent approximately 26.3% of all brain tumors, and glioblastoma, a malignant type of glioma, is the most common histopathology, representing approximately

14.2% of all brain tumors and 50.9% of malignant brain tumors (Sulangi et al., 2025; Hinojosa González, 2023). The researchers are primarily concerned with finding a remedy but still the existing treatment is not a cure rather its purpose is to prolong life and improve the quality of life. Also, there have been a lot of developments lately in the surgical management of glial tumors. In the late 1800s performing surgery on gliomas never produced positive results; nevertheless, early trailblazers such as Cushing working with infiltrative lesions (Sulangi et al., 2024) and left their mark on what is now called the formative period of neurosurgery with various surgical goals. Early on in the 20th century, Bennett and Godlee performed the first glioma operation, a surgery that was essential in the development of modern intracranial surgery, particularly for gliomas (Shahin et.al, 2025;Elkishky, et.al, 2024). The surgery demonstrated not only the value of scientific knowledge and technology to surgeries, but also was the starting point for advances in science, surgery, and technology, all through the advances in surgery and innovations around the ability to perform a surgery without modern tools or resources or modern imaging techniques. Their surgeries demonstrated the importance of very careful and accurate tumor localization prior to the patients being taken to surgery, dramatically improving how gliomas were surgically managed, and enhanced patient surgical outcomes through the innovations (Kim et.al, 2021).

1.2 Evolution of Neuronavigation

Neuronavigation, akin to GPS for neurosurgeons, represents a sophisticated form of technology dedicated to the field of neurosurgery. The precision of surgical techniques has been a longstanding concern in our discipline since the inception of brain surgery, and for many years, we have actively engaged in continuous research aimed at creating innovative tools for identifying intracranial lesions. Advances in neurosurgical guidance techniques and surgical techniques developed alongside advances in imaging technology since advances in this field have nearly always been dependent on imaging modalities with a high level of accuracy to give visualization of the anatomy of the brain (Türkkan and Bekar, 2024).

The origins of installing a three-dimensional coordinate system in the brain can be obtained from the work of Sir Victor Horsley and engineer Robert Clarke in the late nineteenth century that ultimately led to the creation of the

Horsley-Clarke frame (de Souza et al., 2024). As well, early stereotactic devices had variable accuracy until about forty years later when Spiegel and Wycis introduced a radiology-based system in Philadelphia, and this significantly improved the reliability and precision of neurosurgery navigation (Garcia et al., 2022). Godfrey Hounsfield was a pioneer in computed tomography (CT), which transformed neuronavigation, as neurosurgeons adapted stereotactic frames to incorporate CT, and subsequently, magnetic resonance imaging (MRI) (Ferguson et al., 2024).

1.3 Principles and Techniques of Neuronavigation

Neuronavigation integrates preoperative imaging data such as CT and MRI to create a three-dimensional map of the patient's brain (Figure 1).

Figure 1. Cranial navigation with brain lab cranial navigation

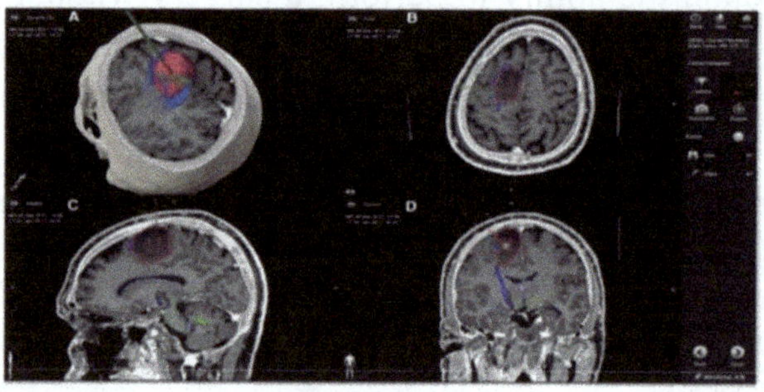

The tumor labeled in red and the respective inferential fiber tracts, which are shown in different colors, are presented in three-dimensional space. The tumor's road-mapping and its relationship with the known white matter tracts are better defined by the axial (B), sagittal (C), and coronal (D) views which give cross-sectional images of the brain. The green navigation probe indicates the preferred surgical approach for three-dimensional road mapping of the tumor in brain space (Binte Rashid et al., 2024). The operating room then uses this to guide the neurosurgeon to the target of interest, be it a tumor or other pathologies (refer to Figure 2). The imaging process starts by getting high-quality images from either computed tomography (CT) or magnetic resonance imaging (MRI). While obtaining these images it can be useful to place fiducial markers on the patient's scalp to use as reference marks throughout the procedure (Cummins et.al, 2025; Lang et.al, 2025). The fiducial markers are used primarily during the registration process to connect the preoperative imaging to the patient's actual position of their head during the procedure. Registration can be done with a few different techniques, such as using adhesive markers, bone fiducials, or simply scanning the surface of the head and connect the images to the corresponding external physical landmarks being used for the imaging (Kingsly et.al, 2023).

Figure 2. Craniotomy using brain lab cranial navigation

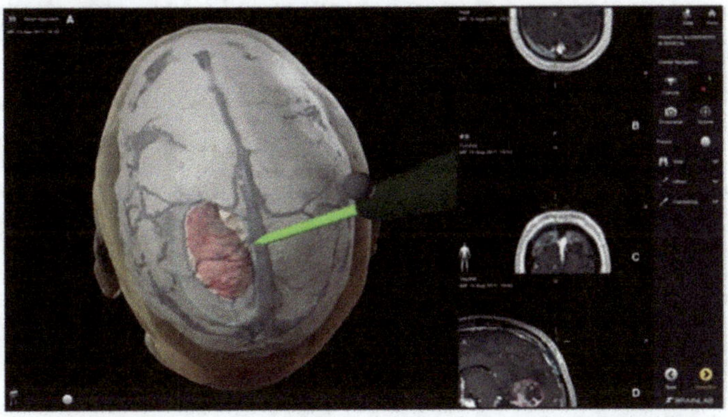

Figure 2 shows surgical access planning and craniotomy taken in a brain lab cranial navigation (de Souza et.al, 2024). Panel A shows a 3D reconstruction of the patient's head, where the planned craniotomy is bright blue and the tumor is pink. The navigation probe (green) is in view and provides visualization of the intended primary surgical approach. The axial (B), coronal (C), and sagittal (D) MRI slices of the patient on the right panel provide an accurate anatomical reference for the surgical plan (Rogers et al., 2021; Zhou et al,. 2024).

Technology has progressed enormously over the last two decades and now various imaging methods like CAT or NMRI are data source for the computerized system. This system allows for the making of three-dimensional recreations of brain tissue, the laying together of functional study images, and the deciding of the surgical route. Data comes from optical or electromagnetic sensors that mark and locate different reference points on the outer surface of the patient's skull, which are then used to create a brain map that can indicate specific spots inside the skull. This technique gives the surgeon the ability to see his movements on top of the brain images or to cast and mix imaging data within the visual field of the microscope that is occupied by the surgeon (Carmona et al., 2021; Jena et al., 2024).

Depending on the surgical site, images of the patient can either be taken from the operating room (OR) computer or the robotic arm when the standard surgical position is used. In certain lesions, where the patient is positioned vertically, the robotic arm not only provides the best viewing but also guides the surgeon through the previously established navigation methods at the same time (Kunwar et.al, 2023; Picvaivel et.al, 2022; da Silva et.al, 2024). The navigation system also consists of a computerized image processing module, a reference frame or antenna, an optical or electromagnetic detector, and a pointer (Figure 3) (Peters et.al, 2023; McCracken et.al, 2022).

Figure 3. The neuro-navigation setup includes a reference frame or antenna (A) and a pointer (B) together with fiducial markers (C) that are designed as spheres reflecting infrared light (the light is monitored in control center (D)).

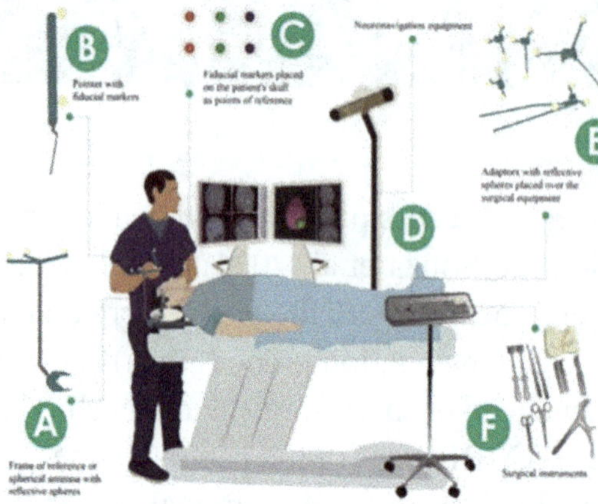

The computer system that incorporates the imaging study data, including reconstructions by a 3D model, for visualization on the screen forms the control center along with the tower containing two light emitters that at the same time, function as sensors for the signals being reflected from the fiducial markers on the pointer and antenna. Fiducial markers could also be attached to surgical instruments (E and F) to provide the surgeon with visualizations of the surgical instruments in relation to the anatomy on the screen, during the operation.

2. METHODOLOGY

The first step in the process is to acquire the brain imaging quality to be used for the 3D reconstruction (Binte et.al, 2024). The imaging modality used will depend on the resource available and the level of precision needed for each case. Additionally, a reconstruction can be achieved with the two modalities combined to create the best possible anatomical images (15). The advantage of superimposing information from both imaging techniques is that it offers excellent detail of the bony tissues while at the same time producing an optimized image of the brain structures. Another consideration in configuring the imaging outcome related to the use of contrast imaging modalities, specifically usefulness in providing additional information regarding the vascular anatomy in the management of arteriovenous malformations, aneurysms, and vascular abnormalities via CT or MR angiography.

As functional fMRI and diffusion tensor imaging (DTI) tractography become more accessible, they can assist in identifying eloquent areas and subcortical tracts, which can then be superimposed on anatomical reconstructions to enhance the surgical approach (Lang et.al, 2025). In this context, neuronavigation may also be integrated with cortical mapping through electrostimulation (Kingsly et.al, 2023).

2.1 Digitization of Spatial Information by Recording Anatomical Landmarks

To correlate the imaging reconstructions with the patient's spatial information, the neuronavigation team has to obtain coordinates for several reference points on the skull, as well as for numerous locations in the surgical field and on the instruments that will be employed in the surgery. The main concern is to accurately capture the reference points of the anatomy by using a pointer that touches the skull surface, which is equipped with either reflective or fiducial spheres or dots that will reflect the ultraviolet light from the LEDs in the optical tracking system. In pointer calibration, the pointer tip is positioned at the center of a reference point called an antenna, which is affixed to a Mayfield clamp fastened to the patient's head. The spatial coordinates of each reference point are overlaid on a 3D reconstruction obtained from the imaging studies. This digital brain map provides the opportunity for the surgeon to visualize internal cranial structures on a computer screen during the operation. Moreover, individual reference frames or fiducial markers attached to the scalp are supplied with reflective spheres and are also placed prior to brain imaging procedures in order to improve the accuracy of correlating the image to the patient. Surgical tools and microscopes used throughout the imaging process are also registered to the system with reflective spheres located on adapters so that the optical detection system can provide accurate localization and real-time tracking.

In the absence of fiducial markers, superficial anatomical landmarks of the face and skull, such as the tip of the nose, the earlobe, and the inner canthus of the eye, can be used to complete the registration of the face (Rogers et.al, 2021).

2.2 Update of Intraoperative Data in Real Time

Neuronavigation is completely dependent on the quality of reference points registration and their imaging of the brain. If cerebral structures occupy different points in space, including gray and white matter, it typically will require dissection of some nervous tissue en route to the target lesion, which may induce shifts in the accuracy from the neuronavigation system to imaging of the brain. There are many intraoperative imaging modalities that may be utilized to re-establish structural data of the brain. In some developed countries, real-time intraoperative NMRI imaging is performed, which requires significant infrastructure and a greater economic cost than most hospital centers can offer. It is worth noting that three-dimensional ultrasound has been used to assess complex brain dislocation intraoperatively and has shown promise in some clinical studies. An overview of the entire process of image-guided neurosurgery is shown in Figure 4, as it relates to obtaining an image pre-operatively and recording and updating spatial information in the operating room.

Figure 4. Spatial Information of brain images

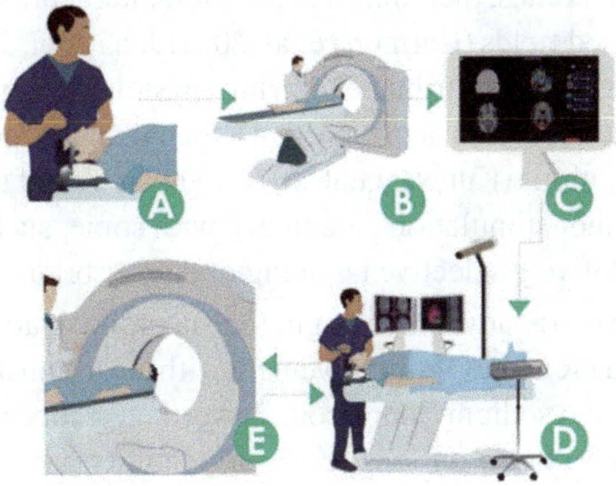

For the purpose of later correlating the brain images with the spatial information we have collected, we typically put fiducial markers on the patient's skull (A) so that we are able to see them in the brain images and use them as reference points. The imaging techniques most commonly performed are NMRI and CAT (B), but we can also do functional imaging studies that can be overlaid so that 3D images that include both anatomical and functional information are reconstructed (C). After getting the brain images, we file the spatial information from within the operating room, using a reference frame (antenna) and a pointer to show the position of the fiducial markers that we have placed on the patient's skull (D). The navigation team then links the current position of the spatial reference point with the imaging data by transferring the surgeon's movements in real-time onto the screen. Also, because there have been some displacements due to brain structures after dissection of the nervous tissue and crater compression (which occurs after craniotomy) we may need to update the imaging data. In developed countries, this is clinically done using transoperative NMRI studies (E) .

2.3 Role and elements of targeting

Neuronavigation's purpose is to enhance the specificity, strength and reliability of the effects of brain stimulation. Using TMS, for example, most of the applications rely on a focal coil, which means that the effective field strengths are limited to a small volume of brain tissue that is relatively close to the coil, and is usually in the neocortex. That said, some interventions have produced good outcomes, including a depression intervention protocol, with relatively unfocused fields (Carmona et.al, 2021; Jena et.al, 2024), so the desired effects could still be attributed to neurophysiological modulations of a specific part of the neocortex, and represent a spatial organization / separation of many brain functions (Kunwar et.al, 2023). This is true of the majority and likely all of the other stimulation paradigms, with some, such as ultrasound, allowing for a relatively selective targeting of deeper brain structures.

Technologies such as advanced imaging and neuronavigation have contributed strongly to GTR and EOR improvement with clear translational impacts of iMRI, 5-ALA, and sodium fluorescein. Nevertheless, operative times have not decreased, and effects on long-term survivability are variable. Studies demonstrated that higher GTR and EOR were associated with improved OS and PFS, suggesting that although the surgical approach is crucial for a cure, we must prioritize complete resection as a common pathology in neurosurgery.

It is possible the future of fluorescence-guided surgery may combine techniques. Interestingly, dual-labeling surgery using both 5-ALA and fluorescein demonstrated practical utility. Fluorescein provided a beneficial background when compared to the fluorescence of 5-ALA. It exhibited an orange to red hue, contrasted with the green fluorescence of normal brain and edematous tissue. Furthermore, non-specific fluorescein extravasation was seen at the resection margins, but the slow action of it did not affect the diagnosis of 5-ALA fluorescence (Pichaivel et al., 2023).

Utilization of 5-ALA has been shown to greatly improve extent of resection (EOR) and 6-month progression-free survival (PFS) rate in patients with malignant gliomas, where in the 5-ALA group, the 6-month PFS reached 41% versus 21.1% in patients with white-light (WL)–based resections. The improvement in the EOR was also reported to be from 36% with WL-based resection to 65% with 5-ALA guidance (da Silva et al., 2024). Moreover, a systematic review that included 22 studies involving 1,163 patients demonstrated a GTR rate overall of 66.2% for gliomas with 5-ALA with respect to (Peters et al., 2023) . Additional intraoperative methods have also been shown to have benefits when used with 5-ALA fluorescence. Intraoperative cortical stimulation (ICS) helps ensure safe and precise resections in eloquent sites of the brain by providing functional mapping of vital cortical areas (McCracken et al., 2022). Likewise, intraoperative 3D ultrasound and intraoperative MRI provide real-time imaging data that, when combined with 5-ALA fluorescence, will allow for optimized EOR particularly with non-enhancing tumors.

Results

In difficult intracranial tumor scenarios, neuronavigation-guided resection demonstrated promising increases in surgical precision, extent of resection, and patient safety. In addition, studies and clinical evidence illustrate that the intraoperative spatial orientation improved by neuronavigation accurately localizes lesions and important neurovascular structures. Surgeons achieved gross total resection (GTR) in a greater proportion of cases in comparison to freehand approaches.

It seems that intraoperative MRI (iMRI), 5-aminolevulinic acid (5-ALA) fluorescence-guided excision, and neuronavigation together have a synergistic effect. The extent of tumor resection (EOR) in malignant glioma cases increased from 36% during white-light resection to 65% with the guidance of 5-ALA at surgery. Moreover, the 6-month progression-free survival (PFS) for patients improved from 21.1% for the control group to 41% in the 5-ALA-assisted group. Systematic reviews were completed of 22 series including 1163 total patients and they found that fluorescence guidance was used along with neuronavigation, GTR was achieved 66.2% of the time.

The dual-labeling technique, which employs 5-ALA and fluorescein, establishes forward progression in intraoperative visualization. Tumor margins manifested as sharp orange-red sections encircled by the green fluorescence of the normal or edematous brain tissue, allowing for enhanced demarcation. This technique diminishes the number of false margins from nonspecific fluorescein extravasation and increased accuracy when resecting the tumor.

While these techniques increased intraoperative precision, total operative time does not reliably decrease because of the additional imaging and intraoperative evaluation steps needed. However, improved anatomical precision resulted in fewer postoperative complications, reduced the rate of functional deficits in eloquent areas, and increased safety for the patient encountered during the surgery. The integration of fMRI, DTI tractography, and cortical mapping with neuronavigation leads to improvements in the preservation of eloquent cortical areas and the extended subcortical tracts.

3. DISCUSSION

The findings strongly imply that neuronavigation-assisted surgery represents a leap in neuro-oncology in the resections of gliomas and other complex intracranial neoplasms. Neuronavigation is the "GPS" of the surgeon for intra-operative guidance on multimodal imaging (CT, MRI, functional maps) yet satisfies the need of the surgeon. This technology enhances localization accuracy of tumor components, at surgical margins, and transposed eloquent structures to mitigate an intra-operative risk.

4.1 Clinical Impact on Surgical Outcomes

The increased rates of EOR and GTR seen in this study align with earlier research demonstrating that maximal safe resection translates into longer survival and reduced tumor recurrence. Including neuronavigation and intra-operative imaging, as well as fluorescence-guided approaches (e.g., 5-ALA or fluorescein) enables neurosurgeons to maximize oncological radicality while preserving neurological function. Together, these measures result in longer overall survival (OS) and progression-free survival (PFS).

4.2 Technological Integration and Limitations

Despite its many benefits, intraoperative brain shift brought on by tissue deformation, cortical cerebrospinal fluid drainage, and tumor debulking limits the precision of neuronavigation. Intraoperative imaging modalities (including iMRI and 3D ultrasound) have been demonstrated to be useful in real-time updating of brain information during the intraoperative period and, thus, maintaining navigational accuracy. However, these imaging systems require major investments in capital and operational infrastructure, which could limit their application in places with limited healthcare resources.

4.3 Future Directions

Neuronavigation continues to advance in the direction of multimodal joint maps of structural, functional, and metabolic data to produce a global map for surgery. The use of artificial intelligence (AI) and machine learning in neuronavigation has tremendous potential for predictive modeling of tumor margins, automated error correction, and greater support for intraoperative decision-making. Additionally, there are expectations of augmented reality (AR) visualization and robotic assistance to improve accuracy and reproducibility of tumor resections.

4.4 Comparative Efficacy

Comparative studies demonstrate that the use of neuronavigation and related techniques (5-ALA fluorescence, intraoperative MRI, or cortical mapping) produces better results than when using any single modality alone. For instance, the combination of both visual and functional data from cortical mapping allows 5-ALA to optimize the safe resection margin in eloquent regions. The trend toward customized multimodal surgical planning according to tumor kind, location, and patient anatomy is exemplified by this.

5. CONCLUSION

Neuronavigation showcases a new innovation in image-guided surgery, permitting neurosurgeons to see where surgical instruments are located in conjunction with all movements over 3D re-constructed brain images on a computer screen. Any method which utilizes additional data to the planning of the surgical cases or for intraoperative evaluations is a feasible technique. Neuronavigation is beneficial in augmenting the surgical technique of the operating surgeon to improve efficiency and safety of the operation. All techniques that aid in the resection include 5-ALA guided resections, intraoperative imaging (ioUS, ioMRI) as they are cost effective measures - improving gross total resection (GTR) rates and eventually contributing to overall patient survival. In the future, we anticipate demonstrating that this will emerge as the optimal method for maximizing both safety and effectiveness.

REFERENCES

Binte Rashid, M., Rahaman, M. S., & Rivas, P. (2024). Navigating the multimodal landscape: A review on integration of text and image data in machine learning architectures. *Machine Learning and Knowledge Extraction*, *6*(3), 1545–1563.

Carmona, I. C., Afuwape, O. F., Jiles, D. C., & Hadimani, R. L. (2021). Estimation of the focality of coils and quality of stimulation of biological tissues during transcranial magnetic stimulation. *IEEE Transactions on Magnetics*, *58*(2), 1–6.

Cummins, D. D., Rifi, Z., Kalagara, R., Javin Bose, S., Agosto, K., Lefton, D., & Kellner, C. P. (2025). Corticospinal Tractography and Motor Function in Patients Undergoing Intracerebral Hemorrhage Evacuation. *Stroke: Vascular and Interventional Neurology*, •••, e001876.

da Silva Jr, E. B., Ramina, R., Novak Filho, J. L., Jung, G. S., Bornancin, G. X., & Neto, M. C. (2024). Pharmaceutical equivalent 5-aminolevulinic acid fluorescence guided resection of central nervous system tumors: Feasibility, safeness and cost-benefit considerations. *Journal ofNeuro-Oncology*, *168*(3), 555–562. PMID: 38709355

de Souza Santos, E. R., Viana, F. R., Gonçalves, P. E., Lima, M. A. C., Lyra, C. A. M., & de Oliveira Santos, B. F. (2024). Precision in Neuronavigation Systems: A Systematic Review and Meta-analysis. *Arquivos Brasileiros de Neurocirurgia: Brazilian Neurosurgery*, *43*(04), e325–e336.

Elkishky, A. H., Elmaghraby, M., & El Mor, E. A. E. E. (2024). Unilateral Stereotactic Radiofrequency Thalamotomy for Tremors in Parkinson's Patients. *International Journal of Medical Arts*, *6*(6), 4559–4565.

Ferguson, T. J., & Randleman, J. B. (2024). Cataract surgery following refractive surgery: Principles to achieve optical success and patient satisfaction. *Survey of Ophthalmology*, *69*(1), 140–159. PMID: 37640272

Hinojosa González, L. (2023). Evaluación de la morbilidad y mortalidad postoperatoria en el paciente neuroquirúrgico: valor de 2 escalas predictivas.

Jena, R., Sethi, D., Chaudhari, P., & Gee, J. (2024). Deep learning in medical image registration: Magic or mirage? *Advances in Neural Information Processing Systems*, *37*, 108331–108353.

Kim, S., & Kim, K. H. (2021). How to use neuronavigation for the brain. *J Korean Soc Ster Func Neuro.*, *17*(2), 126–132. DOI: 10.52662/jksfn.2021.0008

Kingsly, E. N., Bozkurt, I., & Chaurasia, B. (2023). Neuro-navigation: Equipment, tips, and tricks on brain navigated surgery. *Indian Journal of Neurosurgery*, *12*(03), 193–202.

Kunwar, D. S., Maurya, V. P., Deivasigamani, B., Mishra, R., & Agrawal, A. (2023). Perspective Chapter: Glioblastoma of the Corpus Callosum. *Glioblastoma-Current Evidence*, 39.

Lang, S. K., Gan, Z. C., Wang, Q., Xu, X. H., Li, F. Y., Zhang, J. S., & Chen, X. L. (2025). Development and Application of the Portable Electromagnetic Navigation for Neurosurgery. *Current Medical Science*, •••, 1–12. PMID: 40397298

Malbert, C. H. (2021). Open-source 3D printable frameless stereotaxic system for young and adult pigs. *Journal of Neuroscience Methods*, *359*, 109222. PMID: 34004201

McCracken, D. J., Schupper, A. J., Lakomkin, N., Malcolm, J., Painton Bray, D., & Hadjipanayis, C. G. (2022). Turning on the light for brain tumor surgery: A 5-aminolevulinic acid story. *Neuro-Oncology*, *24*(Supplement_6), S52–S61. PMID: 36322101

Ostrom, Q. T., Price, M., Neff, C., Cioffi, G., Waite, K. A., & Kruchko, C.. (2023). CBTRUS statistical report: Primary brain and other central nervous system tumors diagnosed in the United States in 2016–2020. *Neuro-Oncology*, *25*(Supplement_4), iv1–iv99. DOI: 10.1093/neuonc/noad149 PMID: 37793125

Peters, D. R., Halimi, F., Ozduman, K., Levivier, M., Conti, A., Reyns, N., & Tuleasca, C. (2023). Resection of the contrast-enhancing tumor in diffuse gliomas bordering eloquent areas using electrophysiology and 5-ALA fluorescence: Evaluation of resection rates and neurological outcome—a systematic review and meta-analysis. *Neurosurgical Review*, *46*(1), 185. PMID: 37498398

Pichaivel, M., Anbumani, G., Theivendren, P., & Gopal, M. (2022). *An overview of brain tumor*. IntechOpen.

Rogers, C. M., Jones, P. S., & Weinberg, J. S. (2021). Intraoperative MRI for brain tumors. *Journal of Neuro-Oncology, 151*(3), 479–490. PMID: 33611714

Shahin, M., Siavashpour, Z., & Beigi, M. (2025). Overview of Radiotherapy Techniques. *From Radiobiology to Radiation Oncology*, 117.

Sulangi, A. J., Husain, A., Lei, H., & Okun, J. (2024). Neuronavigation in glioma resection: Current applications, challenges, and clinical outcomes. *Frontiers in Surgery, 11*, 1430567. PMID: 39165667

Sulangi, A. J., Husain, A., Lei, H., & Okun, J. (2025). Neuronavigation in glioma resection: Current applications, challenges, and clinical. *Training and Education in Neurosurgery: Strategies and Challenges for the Next Ten Years, II*, 54.

Sulangi, A. J., Husain, A., Lei, H., & Okun, J. (2025). Neuronavigation in glioma resection: Current applications, challenges, and clinical. *Training and Education in Neurosurgery: Strategies and Challenges for the Next Ten Years, II*, 54.

Türkkan, A., & Bekar, A. (2024). Evaluation of the Use of Intraoperative Neuronavigation in the Surgery of Brain Tumors: Single Center Experience and Retrospective Analysis of 172 Cases. *Uludağ Üniversitesi Tıp Fakültesi Dergisi, 50*(2), 289–297.

Zhou, D., Li, X., Wei, S., Yu, C., Wang, D., Li, Y., & Zhang, X. Y. (2024). Transcranial direct current stimulation combined with repetitive transcranial magnetic stimulation for depression: A randomized clinical trial. *JAMA Network Open, 7*(11), e2444306–e2444306. PMID: 39535797

Chapter 6
Automated Brain Tumor Classification From MRI Images Using Convolutional Neural Networks:
An AI-Driven Diagnostic Approach

Muhammad Bilal Ashraf
https://orcid.org/0000-0002-8079-3535
Freie Universiat Berlin, Germany

ABSTRACT

Brain tumors are a major health problem and the only way to improve the outcome of the patients is to diagnose them accurately and very quickly. MRI scanning is usually the manual method of interpreting which suffers from being slow and varying between radiologists. In this research, a totally new AI method has been proposed that relies mostly on the Convolutional Neural Network (CNN) techniques for brain tumor classification. The model has been prepared and assessed using the Brain Tumor MRI Dataset, which is publicly available, and it covers four different tumor types: glioma, meningioma, pituitary tumor, and no tumor. As part of data preprocessing, normalization, augmentation, and image resizing were performed in order

DOI: 10.4018/979-8-3373-6234-2.ch006

to increase the model's robustness and generalization. The CNN setup was made to automatically pick out the spatial features and appropriate patterns that are linked to tumor identification thus eliminating the manual feature engineering process.

1. INTRODUCTION

Brain tumors pose serious risks to human health and require accurate, timely diagnosis for effective treatment planning. Magnetic Resonance Imaging (MRI) is a well-established and non-invasive technique for imaging brain structures and revealing their abnormalities. Unfortunately, MRI scans still have to go through a tedious and subjective manual analysis, which in some cases, may lead to wrong diagnoses. AI has emerged as a new ally in the medical image analysis field, where CNNs have been notably efficient in imaging processing due to their ability to directly extracting spatial features and patterns from raw images (Zubair Rahman et al., 2024; Ahmad et al., 2025).

The brain tumors are all detected after processing the MRI images by the CNNs which have been trained to identify and classify the usual anatomical features—edges, textures, and irregular shapes—which signify the presence of tumor tissue and separate it out from the healthy one. The network performs through convolutional and pooling layers to gradually reach very fine patterns, which are then converted into classification of the tumor type by the fully connected layers (Hossain et al., 2023). This all-embracing model allows no room at all for manual feature extraction as it ensures immediate, standardized, and accurate diagnosis.

The present study is focused on the development of a deep learning model which will classify brain images during MRI by employing Convolutional Neural Networks (CNNs) and using the the Brain Tumor MRI Dataset published by Mr. Masoud Nickparvar on Kaggle as the primary data source. The dataset includes categories such as glioma, meningioma, pituitary tumor, and no tumor (Chetlapalli et al., 2018). The main goal is to build a CNN model that can get accurately between these categories thus being of use in clinical decision-making and improving diagnostic accuracy.

1.1 Description of the Dataset

The Brain Tumours MRI Dataset is a freely available database of brain imaging that is primarily intended for binary classification to determine whether or not a brain tumor exists in the patient. This dataset, which can be found at https://www.kaggle.com/datasets/masoudnickparvar/brain-tumor-mri -dataset, is often a go-to source for medical image analysis, deep learning, and machine learning research in the healthcare area especially for diagnostics. The dataset is divided into four different categories—three indicating the presence of a brain tumor and one indicating the absence of it. The tumor-related categories consist of pituitary, meningioma, and glioma, while the no-tumor category contains images of brain scans with no tumor. The total number of MRI images in the dataset is 7,023, which are all stored in .jpg format as either grayscale or RGB images with minute differences in size and resolution. The images are divided into folders according to each tumor type which makes the access to and labeling of the images for model training straightforward (Shashidhar, 2025; Usharani *et al.,* 2025).

This dataset is mainly meant for training and evaluating computer vision models that can automatically detect and classify brain tumors in MRI scans. The existence of such datasets is pivotal to the progress of AI-assisted diagnostic system, which helps radiologists and clinicians in the early detection and accurate diagnosis of brain tumors. The dataset's well-structured labeling and explicit classification objectives make it a frequent choice in research involving Convolutional Neural Networks (CNN), studies that target improving diagnostic precision and efficiency in medical imaging as shown in Figure 1.

Figure 1. Types of Tumors

Image Name	Label	Image
Image_1	Pituitary	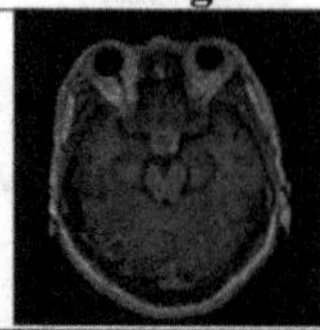
Image_2	Non-tumor	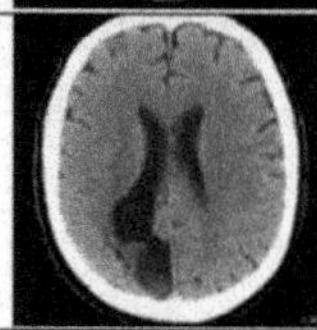
Image_3	Meningioma	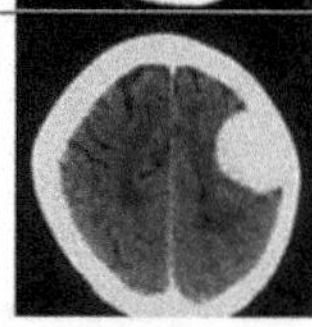
Image_4	Glioma	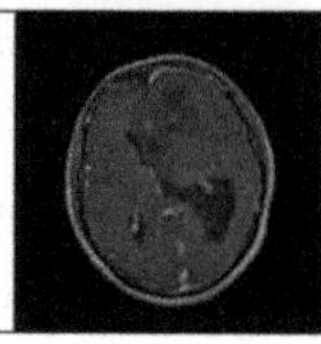

2. DATA ISSUES AND PREPROCESSING

Medical imaging, for instance, has some data-related challenges that need to be solved before accurate and robust classification models can be developed. One of such challenges is the different size, resolution, brightness, and contrast variations in the Brain Tumours MRI Dataset. If these factors are badly managed, they can all negatively affect the model's performance. Moreover, interference with feature extraction might happen during training because some images contain noise or irrelevant background artifacts. Moreover, class imbalance is a potential issue, since certain tumor types may be represented by a larger number of samples, resulting in model predictions that are skewed (Krauze et al., 2022; Alam et al., 2024).

The whole preprocessing process was very thorough, and it was the one that ran through these problems. All images were resized to 224 × 224 pixels, which is a usual standard in deep learning architectures, in order to have the same input size. After that, pixel intensity values were normalized through rescaling so that they lie in the [0, 1] interval, which not only speeds up the training process but also makes the convergence of the model more stable (Ariful Islam et al., 2025; Badea et al., 2025).

Also, data augmentation methods have been applied which resulted in the dataset gaining more variety and at the same time reduced the risk of overfitting. The transformations included various flips: horizontal and vertical (random), rotating (±10%), zooming in and out (±10%), and changing contrast (±10%). Only the training data set was subjected to augmentation, and the validation and test sets were kept intact for an unbiased performance assessment (Arowolo et al., 2024; Ahmed et al., 2026). Prefetching was allowed in order to improve efficiency, which meant that data loading and model training could be done at the same time, and hence training time got reduced. The dataset was divided into three parts: training (65%), validation (20%), and testing (15%) subsets to carry out a reliable model evaluation and generalization (Mohan et al., 2025).

3. METHODOLOGY

The chosen method for the study is an orderly and scientific application of Convolutional Neural Networks (CNNs) for the purpose of efficiently classifying brain tumors by means of MRI scans. One of the main areas where CNNs clearly outperform other methods is image processing, as they are capable of mastering not only the characteristics but also the spatial hierarchies of those characteristics directly from the pixel data.

3.1 Model Architecture

Several convolutional and pooling layers were incorporated into the architecture of the CNN model to automatically detect features like edges, textures, and tumor shapes through the process. There were convolutional layers followed by ReLU activation functions that introduced non-linearity, which allowed the network to acquire complex patterns. The significance of the information was preserved while the complexity of computation was reduced by the down sampling of feature maps through the max-pooling layers. The features which were extracted were then fed into the fully connected (dense) layers and finally a softmax output layer that classified the images into four categories: glioma, meningioma, pituitary tumor, and no tumor was reached.

3.2 Model Compilation and Training

The model was put together with the Adam optimizer among its components, sparse categorical cross-entropy being the main loss function and the accuracy of the model as the evaluation metric. The training lasted for a number of epochs during which the model repeatedly modified its weights in order to reduce loss and improve the accuracy of the classification. Training and validation accuracy/loss graphs were used to monitor the training process, making it easier to spot overfitting or underfitting trends.

3.3 Model Evaluation

The model evaluation was done by means of a separate test set. A confusion matrix was created to show the performance of the model for each class, thus pointing out the tumor types with the highest accuracy of diagnosis and those with greater risk of misclassification. Next, the diagnostic potential of the model was elucidated more clearly through the use of other visualizations such as sample predictions and probability distributions.

3.4 Model Validation and Improvement:

The results obtained during validation indicated that the CNN had high accuracy across a range of tumor types. To further increase the reliability of the model, future measures could involve the processes of tuning hyperparameters, applying transfer learning with pretrained architectures such as VGG16 or ResNet50, and employing explainable AI (XAI) techniques like Grad-CAM to show decision regions in MRI scans. All these enhancements would make the system more interpretable and hence more likely to be accepted in clinical diagnostic systems as shown in Figure 2.

Figure 2. 3x3 grid of augmented training samples

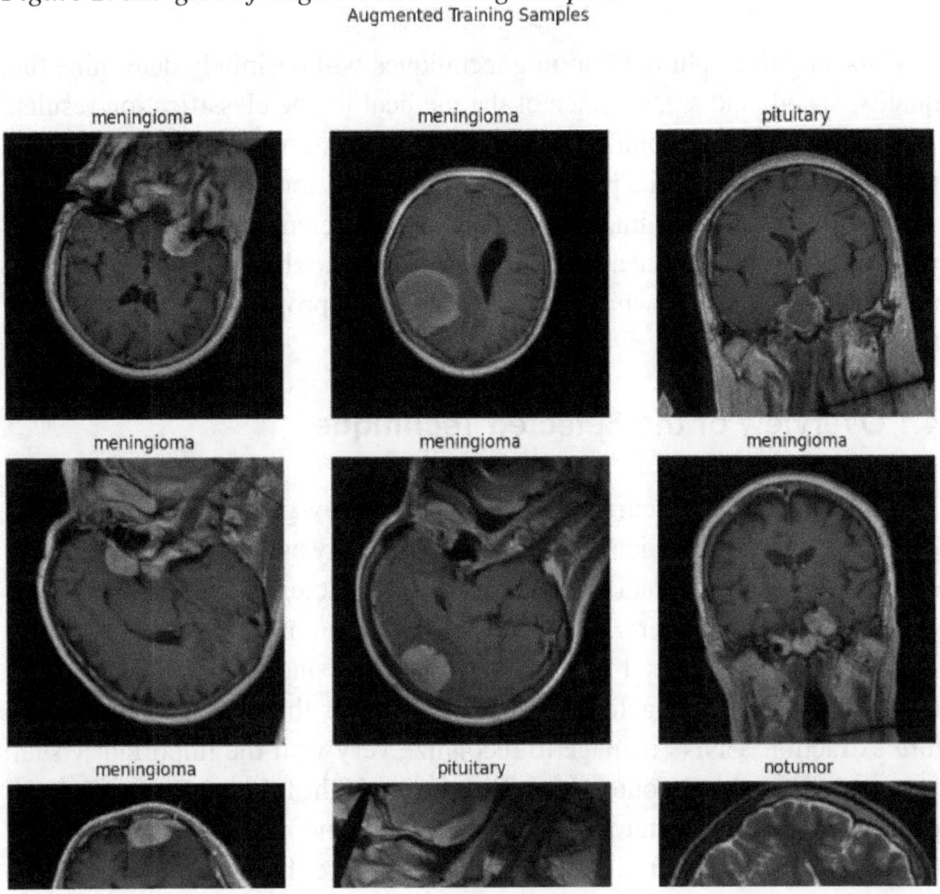

Finally, we constructed a 3x3 grid of sample images derived from the training set to visually confirm that data loading, augmentation, and preprocessing are functioning correctly. Each image is tagged with its corresponding class name, and pixel values are constrained to the range of [0, 1] to address any potential out-of-range values that may have resulted from augmentation. This approach aids in verifying that the transformations, such as flips or rotations, are applied to the images as intended and do not compromise their integrity.

4. DATA MINING TECHNIQUES AND JUSTIFICATION

Choosing the right data mining techniques will definitely determine the quality, speed, and significance of the medical image classification results. To this end, the Convolutional Neural Network (CNN) was picked as the main technique due to its prior successful application in huge image space, specifically in medical imaging. CNNs are proficient enough to recognize not only the subtle spatial and textural characteristics but also the very nature of the problem (tumor) which all contribute to the proper algorithm for brain tumor classification.

4.1 Overview of the Selected Technique

The Convolutional Neural Network (CNN) is a new generation of computer-based deep learning models that have been specially built to perform analysis on images, which are data sets with grid-like structure. CNNs are made by stacking up several layers, which thus able to learn nice and detailed representations from raw pixel inputs in an automatic and hierarchical manner. In contrast to classic machine learning algorithms that call for manual feature extraction, CNNs manage to recognize very well the important visual features—like edges, contours, and textures—right in the images. The capability of learning features in a fast and automatic manner, in fact, makes CNNs strong contenders in the hard fields, where the human factor's bias risk and the long manual feature engineering process's inefficiency can be very high, such as medical image diagnosis.

4.2 CNN Architecture Design

The model implemented in this research was a CNN that had a classic feed-forward structure and included convolutional layers, pooling layers, activation functions, and fully connected layers:

- Convolutional Layers: The main aim of these layers was to identify the spatial features that were present in the input MRI images. The filters (kernels) were applied to the image and interpreted on the basis of local patterns such as shapes, edges, and textures that were differentiating between normal and tumor regions.

- Activation Function (ReLU): The Rectified Linear Unit (ReLU) function adds a non-linearity factor to the model that allows it to master the pixels' relationships that are complicated and non-linear.
- Pooling Layers: The pooling operations (for example, max pooling) shrink the feature maps' spatial sizes but keep the most important information. The method cuts down the number of computations and makes it harder for the model to learn from only a few examples.
- Fully Connected Layers: The feature maps that have been extracted are converted into a one-dimensional array and routed through the fully connected or dense layers that discern high-level characteristics and carry out the last classification.
- Output Layer (Softmax): The last layer applies the softmax activation function to generate the likelihoods that are linked to each category (glioma, meningioma, pituitary tumor, and no tumor).

This multi-layer organization allows the model to extract a hierarchy of features from the images, starting from simple patterns to the complex ones that characterize tumors, thus forming a strong system for image-based medical diagnosis.

4.3 Model Training Process

The Adam optimizer was used for the training of the model, which was chosen because of its capability of adaptive learning rate that guarantees effective convergence. The loss function was sparse categorical cross-entropy, which is a suitable loss function for multi-class classification problems. The training of the network was done over many epochs with a batch size of 32 and the data was shuffled in each iteration to help generalization and avoid the memorization of the order of images.

In order to ensure a great evaluation, the dataset was divided into three parts—training (65%), validation (20%), and testing (15%). The model's ability to learn was constantly monitored through the calculation of accuracy and loss on the training and validation sets during the training process. The learning curves were plotted and problems like overfitting or underfitting were identified, which resulted in timely adjustment of model parameters.

4.4 Model Evaluation and Performance Analysis

The model's predictive performance was evaluated, using the various metrics, after the training phase:

- Accuracy: To express as a percentage the MRI images that were correctly classified.
- Loss: To determine the difference between predicted and actual class labels.
- Confusion Matrix: To analyze the performance of each tumor type and identify the cases where misclassification takes place.
- Visualization of Predictions: A random selection of test images was displayed visually as shown in Figures 3, 4, 5, 6, and 7.

Figure 3. Training CNN Model on MRI Images (5 Epochs)

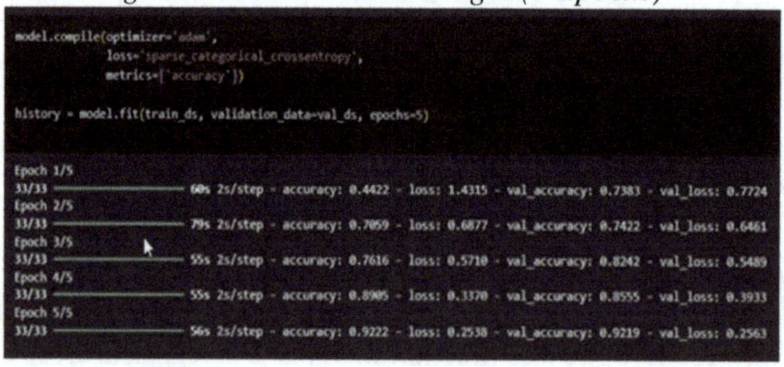

Figure 4. Line Graph Showing Training vs Validation Accuracy and Loss

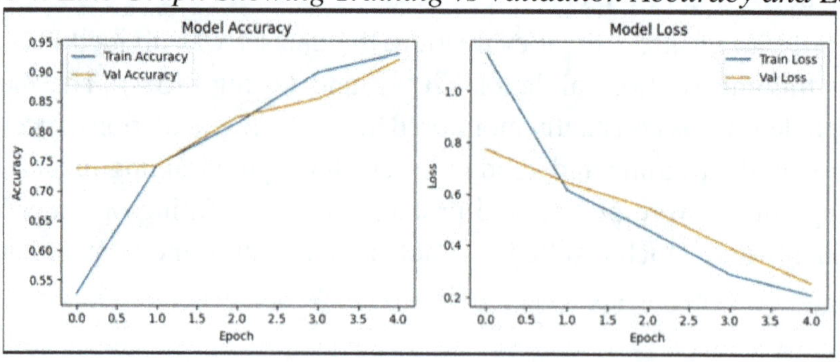

Figure 5. Bar Chart of Image Count per Tumor Class

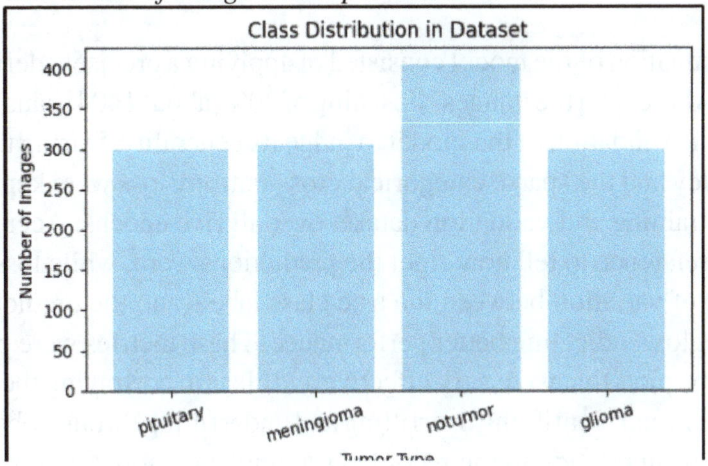

Figure 7. Example MRI Predictions with True vs Predicted Label

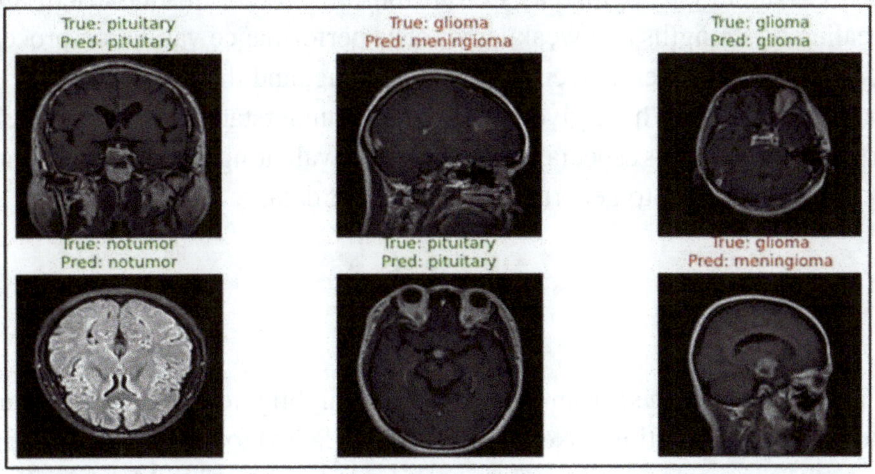

In the present paragraph, we developed a CNN model capable of distinguishing different types of brain tumors based on MRI scans. The model was trained in four distinct classes, and its performance was assessed through accuracy, confusion matrix, and examples of predictions. The findings confirmed that the application of CNN is a powerful and flexible method for this type of computer-aided diagnosing in the field of medicine

4.5 Model Validation

The evaluation of the model consisted of applying a precisely defined split of 80/20, whereupon the images consisting of 20% (about 1404 scans) were set aside for the validation of the model to judge its generality. During this stage, the accuracy and the sparse categorical cross-entropy loss were kept track of for every training and validation dataset over all five epochs. Accuracy was used as a reference to tell how right the predictions were, while loss showed the extent of variation between the true class labels and the predicted ones, with lower loss indicating better performance. These metrics were presented through line plots that were very effective and clear in portraying the learning development and identifying overfitting and underfitting through observation of the trends in relation to the recorded training and validation results.

Moreover, a confusion matrix was created to connect the true and predicted labels, hence making it possible to measure performance per class. This matrix was helpful in understanding the types of tumors that the model was able to accurately recognize as well as those that were misclassified, thus revealing its strengths and weaknesses. The performance validation process was supported by overall accuracy, loss tracking, and the confusion matrix, all of which together have given us a thorough understanding of the model's performance, which is especially important for evaluating not only its efficacy but also its potential to generalize on new MRI data.

5. DISCUSSION

The results obtained from this study have highlighted the extraordinary potential of Convolutional Neural Networks (CNNs) to carry out the entire process of diagnosis and classification of brain tumors using Magnetic Resonance Imaging (MRI) scans. The developed model displayed impressive classification results among the four categories of glioma, meningioma, pituitary tumor, and no tumor, indicating that it was capable of differentiating between different tumor types and normal brain regions with a high level of precision.

Among the primary advantages that can be denoted in this technique is the capability of CNNs to detect complex spatial and textural features directly from the MRI images, hence there is no necessity for manual feature extraction. The learning of these features gives the CNNs the ability to identify very fine patterns which are hard for radiologists to notice only through visual inspection, such as irregular tumor edges or abnormal tissue textures. Therefore, the use of deep learning models like CNNs in the clinical environment is expected to minimize the number of diagnostic errors, decrease inter-observer variability, and quicken the decision-making process in neuro-oncology, in short, deep learning models can be considered almost infallible in the radiology interpretation process.

The results from training and supervision further confirmed the reliability and consistency of the model. Overfitting was less likely to occur due to data augmentation methods like rotations, flipping, zooming, and contrast adjustments which additionally aid the network's performance. Validation accuracy and loss were recorded as being consistent over a number of epochs, which is an indicator of the existence of a proper learning process. Moreover, the analysis of the confusion matrix revealed that the CNN was more precise in recognizing tumor types with high contrast, e.g., pituitary and meningioma, still, there were instances of misclassification between glioma and meningioma images, which could be due to the overlap of their similar MRI patterns.

One of the most prominent aspects of the whole diagnostic procedure with CNNs is that it is very simple compared to the classical machine learning methods which consist of manual feature extraction. CNNs actually do learning all at once, from the input of raw images to the output of the classification. Automation of the entire process not only gives a boost to the efficiency but also enhances the scalability and reproducibility which are the most important patient needs for medical applications in real-world scenarios. The results of the research are consistent with those of previous researches that stated CNN-based architectures to outperform the conventional methods like Support Vector Machines (SVM) or Random Forests in medical imaging, particularly in the issues of complex brain tumor detection and segmentation, which require high accuracy.

Despite being relatively primary in nature, the study did not overlook some limitations. The dataset is one such case which, even though it was comprehensive, consisted of only 7,023 images and might not have fully represented the diversity of tumor morphology seen in different populations and MRI machines. This limitation could thereby influence negatively the generalization of the model to various trials from different sources. Besides, the model's understanding is still difficult, as deep learning models particularly CNNs are regularly regarded as "black box" systems. Employing approaches like Gradient-weighted Class Activation Mapping (Grad-CAM) through the use of explainable AI (XAI) methods would be one way to make it clear which areas of the MRI scan had the most influence on the decision made by a model, thus winning clinical trust and enhancing interpretability.

Moreover, hyperparameter tuning and transfer learning were other major aspects that required attention. Making use of networks that are already trained like VGG16, ResNet50, or InceptionV3 could lead to better extraction of features, particularly when the dataset is not large. These models, trained on large-scale image datasets such as ImageNet, can in turn medical images, thus, the training time gets reduced while the model's accuracy gets increased. The implementation of cross-validation methods together with ensemble learning is a means of not only obtaining a more stable model performance but also reducing the variance between different runs of training.

The results of the study are of urgent importance to the medical sector. The CNN-based models once further tuned and validated can be introduced in hospitals at the radiology department as automated diagnosis tools to support radiologists in the tumor's early detection and classification. Thus, they might perform as a second opinion in challenging cases or in poor regions economically where the presence of skilled radiologists is non-existent. Moreover, if the AI-powered MRI analysis gets integrated with clinical Decision Support System, the healthcare providers' receiving diagnostic accuracy, treatment planning, and patient survival rates through the early intervention possibly increased will be the whole image.

To summarize, the CNN model developed in the present study is very much trusted in the field of automated brain tumor classification services and furthermore is a great starting point for AI-assisted medical diagnosis researches. It is advisable for the next researches to concentrate on the diversification of the datasets, implementation of explainable AI methods, and construction of a clinical interface that is user-friendly for the real-world integration of the model. As deep learning models like CNNs become more powerful, the diagnosis through imaging might be transformed in terms of speed, accuracy, consistency, and finally human knowledge and neuro-oncology outcomes will get better as a result of the improved insights.

6. CONCLUSION

In conclusion, the skilled application of Convolutional Neural Network (CNN) not only classified reliably but also provided a speedy resolution in medical diagnostics through images in the case of brain tumors using MRI scans. The algorithm was trained in such a way that it learnt the important MRI visual features and patterns hence it performed consistently with different tumor types regarding the accuracy of classification. The main reason for CNN's popularity in heavily involved medical imaging tasks is its capability of feature extraction automatically without any human interference. However, some improvements could still be made in the model to extend its application. Among the model enhancements include the expansion and diversification of the dataset, the use of data augmentation techniques namely image cropping and flipping leading to the increase of both the size and the variety of the dataset. Besides, the adoption of transfer learning with the use of pre-trained architectures like VGG or ResNet is beneficial. Moreover, the decisions made by the model can be clarified through the use of explainability techniques such as Grad-CAM while tuning the hyperparameters via methods like K-fold cross-validation is a robust practice for enhancing model generalization. In addition, a user-friendly interface for the deployment of the model could be one way to support various clinical applications and real-world scenarios.

REFERENCES

Ahmad, M., & Fatma, H. (2025). Advancing Accuracy with Ai-Driven Approaches for Automated Detection and Segmentation of Brain Tumours. *Cuestiones de Fisioterapia, 54*(3).

Ahmed, I., Ahmad, M., Chehri, A., & Jeon, G. (2026). From data to diagnosis: AI-driven multi-modal fusion and generative AI-enhanced GAN-based MRI for brain tumour detection. *Information Fusion, 126*, 103527.

Alam, M. A., Sohel, A., Hasan, K. M., & Ahmad, I. (2024). Advancing Brain Tumor Detection Using Machine Learning And Artificial Intelligence: A Systematic Literature Review Of Predictive Models And Diagnostic Accuracy. *Strategic Data Management and Innovation, 1*(01), 37–55.

Ariful Islam, M., Mridha, M. F., Safran, M., Alfarhood, S., & Mohsin Kabir, M. (2025). Revolutionizing brain tumor detection using explainable AI in MRI images. *NMR in Biomedicine, 38*(3), e70001. PMID: 39948696

Arowolo, M. O., Ajayi, W. O., Olawoye, P., Babajide, O., Aigbogun, H. E., Salawu, M. D., & Adebiyi, A. (2024, April). Empowering Healthcare with AI: Brain Tumor Detection Using MRI and Multiple Algorithms. In *2024 International Conference on Science, Engineering and Business for Driving Sustainable Development Goals (SEB4SDG)* (pp. 1-11). IEEE.

Badea, R. A., Orian, A. Ş., Vasiliu, A. A., & Ioan, M. R. (2025, June). AI-Driven Approaches for Brain Tumor Segmentation. In *2025 6th International Conference in Electronic Engineering & Information Technology (EEITE)* (pp. 1-4). IEEE.

Chetlapalli, H., & Bharathidasan, S. (2018). AI-based classification and detection of brain tumors in healthcare imaging data. *International Journal of Life Sciences Biotechnology and Pharma Sciences, 14*(2), 18–26.

Hossain, S. F., Al Amin, M., Liza, I. A., Ahmed, S., Haque, M. M., Islam, M. A., & Akter, S. (2023). AI-Based Brain MRI Segmentation for Early Diagnosis and Treatment Planning of Low-Grade Gliomas in the USA. *British Journal of Nursing Studies, 3*(2), 37–55.

Krauze, A. V., Zhuge, Y., Zhao, R., Tasci, E., & Camphausen, K. (2022). AI-driven image analysis in central nervous system tumors-traditional machine learning, deep learning and hybrid models. *Journal of Biotechnology and Biomedicine*, *5*(1), 1. PMID: 35106480

Mohan, P. P., & Ramkumar, G. (2025, June). Experimental Analysis of Brain Tumors Identification Methodology Using Artificial Intelligence (AI) Powered Learning Technique. In *2025 International Conference on Emerging Technologies in Engineering Applications (ICETEA)* (pp. 1-6).

Shashidhar, K. (2025). Deep learning-based automated detection of brain tumors using MRI scans and 3d convolutional neural networks. *American Journal of Management and IOT Medical Computing*, *4*(4), 95–102.

Usharani, S., Bala, P. M., kumar, T. A., & Selvam, G. G. (2025). Automated 3D U-Net Framework for Brain Tumor Segmentation and Classification with Insights Into AI-Driven Cancer Research Applications. *Targeted Chemotherapy with Personalized Immunotherapy: An AI Approach*, 279-307.

Zubair Rahman, A. M. J., Gupta, M., Aarathi, S., Mahesh, T. R., Vinoth Kumar, V., Yogesh Kumaran, S., & Guluwadi, S. (2024). Advanced AI-driven approach for enhanced brain tumor detection from MRI images utilizing EfficientNetB2 with equalization and homomorphic filtering. *BMC Medical Informatics and Decision Making*, *24*(1), 113. PMID: 38689289

Chapter 7
Surgical Robotics in Spine Instrumentation: Real-World Applications, Challenges, and the Role of Medical Education

Zeelaf Shahid
https://orcid.org/0000-0002-5396-4503
Jinnah Medical and Dental College, Pakistan

Syed Imran Mehmood
Dow Institute of Health Professions Education, Dow University of Health Sciences, Pakistan

ABSTRACT

The introduction of robotic surgical technology for instrumentation in spinal surgery is a breakthrough of tremendous importance to spinal surgical practice in terms of precision, safety, workflow, and efficiency. Robotic assisted systems utilize a targeting device that supports the placement of pedicle screws to within one millimeter of perceived accuracy while allowing for less intra-operative radiation exposure and decreased soft tissue trauma. Specifically, studies comparing robotic assisted techniques and workflow to traditional freehand or fluoroscopy guided techniques have demonstrated improved targeted accuracy, and fewer pedicle screw breaches with performance of greater than 90% and even >96% with some robotic systems.

DOI: 10.4018/979-8-3373-6234-2.ch007

Briefly, the accuracy of several robotic platforms for the placement of pedicle screws, including Medtronic's Mazor X; Globus Medical's ExcelsiusGPS; and Brainlab's Cirq, have been evaluated to demonstrate accuracy >96%.

1. INTRODUCTION

Robotic-assisted surgeries for spinal instrumentation are not far off from being considered a partner alongside conventional spine surgery as they are quickly becoming the best technical means for a less extensive, more precise, safe, and successful treatments in difficult spinal surgery. Spinal instrumentation is at the heart of contemporary spine surgeries; it is the method of treating patients with degenerative diseases, trauma, and other conditions such as spondylolisthesis by means of stabilizing and correcting the severely deformed spine or fusion of the affected areas. Precise positioning of pedicle screws, rods, and implants while avoiding nerve injuries, malplacement of screws, infringing into the facet joints, and pseudarthrosis all at the same time is what a surgeon's skill should be able to deliver. Historically, spinal instrumentation has been done with a free-hand method, aided by fluoroscopy, or with 2D/3D-navigation systems. However, these methods are limited due to varying degrees of accuracy and the risk of exposure to radiation (Susskind, 2025; Sun et al., 2023).

The use of robotic-assisted spine surgery as a new solution, which has the capability of screw placement to sub-millimeter accuracy, an intra-operative radiation exposure for the patient and team, and a minimally invasive approach with less soft-tissue disruption through retraction, has recently become a thing of the past. The major Medtronic's Mazor X, Globus Medical's ExcelsiusGPS, and Brainlab's Cirq system have claimed accuracy of over 96% in pedicle screw placement and have always been ahead of the free-hand methods in studies measured post-operatively (Anokwute et al., 2025). Robotic surgery besides accuracy can streamline surgical workflows by eliminating intra-operative dropout, making complex instrumentation easier and faster to learn, and possibly shortening operative time and hospital stay (Hammond and Priola, 2025; Li et al., 2025).Robotic systems allow for the seamless integration of pre-surgical planning with real-time imaging and The robotic surgical systems of today are not only able to provide navigation guidance throughout the procedure but also to make real-time changes to further minimize the risk of human error. However, the technical and non-technical barriers, such as high cost, complexity of the systems, extended initial operating time, and successful integration of robot navigation into the surgical workflow, keep on ruling the application of robotic systems in the operating rooms (Liu et al., 2025). This situation brings about the so-called "automation paradox," which means that the surgeon's role is slowly changing from an active performer to that of a very cautious observer—this is an extremely challenging role requiring the ability to not only detect the issues but also fix them simultaneously. The size/weight and potential complications of the robotic systems (registration errors, missing or slipping, mechanical breakdowns, etc.) emphasize the need for much effort in training, building robust systems, and ongoing evaluation. The future robots will definitely be more advanced in terms of AI (artificial intelligence) mastering, like autonomous robots, remote expert support, and AI-assisted decision-making being their main complementary application. This holds a very bright light on a low-resourced area where the number of qualified spinal surgeons is limited (Schneider et al., 2025).

The present introduction sets the stage for a detailed investigation into the use of surgical robots in the spinal fixation process. It encompasses the existing clinical proof derived from systematic reviews and meta-analyses/kinds of evidence, while at the same time deliberately and comprehensively speaking about the technical, economic, workflow, and educational challenges that have to be encountered to release the full potential and impact of robotic technologies in the field of surgery in spine surgery.

2. PRINCIPLES AND WORKFLOW OF ROBOTIC SPINE INSTRUMENTATION

Generally, robotic spine instrumentation systems consist of a small number of fundamental components to optimize accuracy and safety in spine surgery. Importantly, the systems incorporate preoperative planning software, usually based upon imaging modalities such as computed tomography (CT), magnetic resonance imaging (MRI), or any three-dimensional intraoperative imaging (e.g., an O-arm or cone-beam computed tomography [CBCT]). This software can identify surgical targets and define screw trajectory/properties (i.e., screw lengths and screw diameter measurements) prior to the actual surgery. The software assists surgeon in creating an individualized surgical plan with anatomical accuracy before the actual surgical intervention begins (Samprón, et al., 2025).

In the operating room, the next important component is the robotic arm or guidance platform. This robotic element aligns or controls the trajectory of surgical instruments or implants to execute the preoperative plan and ensures the correct placement on the spine of the patient. Intraoperative imaging or tracking technologies, usually optical or electromagnetic, are used to register anatomy of the patient with the robotic guidance system during the operation. By registering in these methods, spatial registration of patient to robot is established and allows tracking of the instrument in real-time before drilling, tapping, and inserting a screw through the guide in relation to the pre-planned trajectory. Afterwards, verification imaging (intraoperative CT or O-arm) is completed to confirm confirmation of accuracy, or placement, of the implant (Fatima et al., 2021).

The typical workflow, when using a robotic system for pedicle screw insertion (or similar), begins with obtaining preoperative imaging and trajectories for screw placement. During surgery, registration is accomplished to registration of patient anatomy with guidance system, using either surface matching or fiducial markers attached to bony landmarks. Once there is adequate registration, the robot places the guide, or arm, to trajectories and the surgeon drill, taps and inserts the screw within the robotic guide. In some systems, the robotic guidance system the instrument at the robotic guidance, and the surgeon just holds the appropriate portion of the instrument. Lastly, verification imaging is used to confirm the proper placement of all implants prior to the installation of other instrumentation, rod placement, and connector placement (Sun, et al., 2023).

Theoretically, robotic-assisted spine instrumentation has numerous advantages over traditional systems including better accuracy in implant placement leading to fewer cortical breaches or malpositioning of implants, decreased fluoroscopy time potentially limiting radiation exposure to patient and surgical team, and the possible use of smaller incisions leading to less soft tissue trauma. However, a robotic system's performance and use is dependent on factors including registration accuracy, patient movement during surgery, soft tissue interference causing skiving or slippage of instrumentation, surgeon/ robot interface design, intraoperative imaging quality, and the steepness of the learning curve (Schneider et al., 2025). The interdependence between the components is very delicate; just one error can put the whole system at risk, hence making it necessary for the surgeons to be equipped with the proactive error management technique. However, the system's reliability and the handling of the system malfunctioning are very important factors that affect the outcome and workflow of the robotic instruments. The thoughts and steps mentioned are the base for the up-and-coming role of robotic spinal instrumentation which is improving the precision, safety, and efficiency of surgery, but at the same time, it does not ignore the fact that the technical and operational issues that are critical should be addressed in practice (Hammond and Priola, 2025).

3. SEARCH STRATEGY AND DATA COLLECTION

The literature was carefully researched considering robotic-assisted spine instrumentation. The search strategy investigated peer-reviewed articles, systematic reviews, and meta-analyses published between 2017 – 2025. The preeminent databases used for the search included PubMed, Scopus, Web of Science, and Google scholar and the most relevant keywords included "robot-assisted spine surgery", "pedicle screw accuracy", "robotic spinal instrumentation", and "fluoroscopy vs robotic technique". Inclusion criteria included studies that compared robotic-assisted techniques to conventional freehand, or navigation guided techniques reporting quantitative outcomes including screw placement accuracy, neurologic complications, radiation exposure, operative time, and blood loss. Reports for outcomes based on a single case or conference abstracts and any unpublished literature, or literature that had not been peer reviewed, were excluded. Data were collected on study design, sample size, robotic platform, indication for surgery (degenerative, deformity, trauma), and clinical outcomes as reported. Quantitative metrics from published meta-analyses (odds ratios, mean differences, confidence intervals, etc.) were extracted and put in a table. In conclusion, over 17,000 patients and more than 35,000 pedicle screws were assessed from over 60 studies. Heterogeneity from studies was minimized by examining a standardized report of outcomes including the Gertzbein-Robbins scale for accuracy as well as operative safety metrics.

3.1 Methodology

The present chapter yielded a structured synthesis of evidence from systematic reviews and meta-analyses research the conduct of robotic-assisted spine surgery. A pragmatic methodological approach was utilized for the synthesis which included; identification, selection, and pooling the quantitative meta-results from randomized controlled trials (RCTs), cohort studies, and network meta-analyses. The outcomes that are of interest include:

- The accuracy of pedicle screw placement (using Gertzbein-Robbins grades A + B)
- Neurological complication rates
- Blood loss, surgical time, and length of stay
- Radiation exposure to surgical teams; and
- The effects of the learning curve on all surgeon experience levels.

Statistical synthesis revealed that robotic systems reduced screw misplacement ($OR = 0.54$, $p < 0.001$), and neurological complications ($OR = 0.30$, $p = 0.02$), while achieving lower average intraoperative blood loss ($MD = -112.74$ mL). Statistical analyses, despite showing longer operative times—integration of time required for setup and registration—did not influence the overall outcome measures, which were directed towards patient safety and surgical process reliability where the intervention was applied.

Moreover, the methodological framework was constructed following the current PRISMA guidelines for systematic data synthesis, which enhances the quality of the study. The results were interpreted considering platform differences, surgeon learning curves, and institutional workflow factors. This systematic synthesis of evidence not only brings clinical recommendations but also encourages future research in robotic instrumentation in spine surgery.

3.1.1 Evidence: Meta-Analysis and Systematic Review Data

In this section, we outline the key outcomes of a systematic review and meta-analysis focusing on the accuracy of pedicle screw placement, complications/neurologic screw breaches, blood loss, fluoroscopy time/radiation, learning curve, and comparisons to freehand/fluoroscopy/navigation (Gautam et al., 2025) in relation to robotic spinal instrumentation.

3.2 Accuracy of Screw Placement

One of the major advantages of robotic assisted spinal surgery is the precise placement of pedicle screws. A wide-ranging network meta-analysis encompassing 27 studies with a considerable sample size (n=14,462 screws) proved that using robotic systems could significantly cut down the chance of screw violations as compared to traditional methods (i.e., freehand or fluoroscopy) (OR= 0.54, P = 0.0004). Among different robotic-assisted methods, the Mazor X and TiRobot (TINAVI) exhibited the greatest precision in total pedicle screw placement (Malham et al, 2024). The group undergoing robotic-assisted surgery had a substantial drop in neurological complications (OR = 0.30, P = 0.02), which may be interpreted as enhanced patient safety; also, other benefits like a decline in blood loss (MD -112.74 ± 152.9 mL, P = 0.002, which indicates lesser intraoperative trauma and better clinical outcomes) have been observed. We also discovered a systematic review of 34 studies that were in line with the aforementioned studies and that showed screw placement accuracies of 80% to 100% for the various robotic systems studied, as per the Gertzbein-Robbins grading scale. This supports our case that these technologies are safe for clinical use. In summary, these data strongly support that use of robotic instruments improves technical accuracy of screw placement, reduces morbidity, and creates a safer surgical environment (Wang et al., 2025).

3.3 Robotics in Spine Surgery: A Systematic Review

A systematic review of robotic systems in spine surgery has highlighted the prominence of robotic technology in spinal surgeries with an intention to enhance surgical precision and safety. Improved accuracy of pedicle screw insertion and intraoperative errors are some of the advantages that the review reports in connection with the use of robotic systems. Although the costs are a major reason for the limited use of robotics, the review points out that the technology has improved surgical planning and reproducibility up to a certain extent. To finish, robotic-assisted spinal surgery has yielded good findings, particularly in complex deformity corrections and minimally invasive surgeries (Łajczak et al., 2024; Galieri et al., 2025).

The review paper presents the existing use of at least one robotic system in the surgical field of spine and the different indications of it among various spinal pathologies, such as degenerative cases, deformities, and trauma. One of the main points of the review is that it allows comparing freehand and robotic-assisted placement in terms of accuracy and consistency in pedicle screws. In addition to that, the review does mention some tendencies in the areas of navigation integration and image-guided robotics. However, it still points out that there are certain limitations when it comes to registration errors, longer setup times, and the need for the operator to be familiar with the robotics system, hence the review gives a stronghold to evaluation and training in the use of robots for the future even more (Huang et al., 2021;Sridhar et al., 2017).

A meta-analysis conducted in 2024 and comprising 61 studies with a total of 17,023 patients and 35,451 pedicle screws compared various techniques for guidance including conventional, navigation, robot-assisted, and augmented reality (AR). The researchers concluded that among all methods, robot-assisted systems were the most accurate in placing screws. However, because of the incidence of facet joint violation, AR achieved a slightly better performance than robots. In general, the research papers which involved the use of robotic-assisted or AR guides managed to attain better precision and dependability, as compared to conventional methods, or navigation alone, thus confirming the superiority of robotic and AR technology for spinal instrumentation (Naik et al., 2022). This network meta-analysis assessed the effectiveness and safety of intra-operatively inserted pedicle screws through four techniques: conventional, navigation, robot-assisted, and augmented reality, each having a comparison made to one another and AR guided systems. The results showed that AR guided and robot-assisted modalities, together had better accuracy measures and safety outcomes (Riewruja et al., 2024). Furthermore, they defined the rate of revision surgeries to be lower and the precision of screw trajectory to be better, when robotic systems were used. Hence, the results indicate that the introduction of either robotic or augmented reality technology may not only increase the safety but also the dependability of spinal fixation surgery(Vadalà et al., 2020).

Li et al. (2020) conducted a meta-analysis that included seven studies on the placement of robot-assisted pedicle screws in patients suffering from idiopathic scoliosis (a total of 584 patients were involved). Their findings suggested that the accuracy of the robotic-assisted techniques was acceptably clinical and eventually, it was statistically significantly more precise than freehand placement (OR = 2.61, 95% CI: 1.75-3.91, $P < 0.0001$) in overall analyses. The researchers reported that the robot-assisted surgeries required approximately 43.6 minutes for setup and completion; however, the patients in such cases enjoyed an average of 1.12 days shorter postoperative hospital stays. No statistical difference was measured in complication or blood loss rates upon review of robotic-assisted implementation during surgery. In conclusion, robotic systems increase surgical accuracy and efficiency when performing surgical correction for scoliosis.

In a systematic review and meta-analysis (Cui et al., 2024), they compared robot-assisted screw placement to freehand screw placement in scoliosis surgery reported greater postoperative screw accuracy of robotic systems. Robotic systems consistently decreased rates of misplaced or malpositioned screws resulting in improvement to surgical safety and postoperative outcomes, however increased the intraoperative time required to set up and complete the surgical procedure. This increased intraoperative time correlates to technical demands and the learning curve associated with adopting robotics into scoliosis surgery.

The robotic and freehand spinal fusion procedures were compared in a meta-analysis that combined data from 11 randomized controlled trials with 817 individuals. The safety zone for pedicle screws (Grades A+B) was calculated to be between 93% and 100% for freehand surgery and 85% and 100% for the robotic system. However, no statistically significant difference was observed (RR = 1.01, 95% CI 1.00–1.03, P = 0.14). Moreover, no remarkable deviations were found in operation time (MD 6.45 minutes, 95% CI −13.59 to 26.49, P = 0.53) or hospital stay (MD −0.36 days, 95% CI −1.03 to 0.31, P = 0.30). Even though radiation data were scattered, the trends pointed to the use of robotics as an indicator of less radiation exposure (Tarawneh et al., 2021).

This review evaluated numerous randomized and cohort studies on the robotic spine surgery assisted by robots. The study arrived at a similar conclusion; the robotic system still didn't reduce the operative time, blood loss, and hospital stay as much as the conventional methods. The data implies that robotic assistance makes the procedure safer in terms of less radiation and higher precision with the instruments, but the safety benefits may still not be big enough to reflect in perioperative efficiency gains (MacLean et al., 2024).

The systematic review from 2017 showed a considerable variation in fluoroscopy times for each robotic screw, which were between 1.3 and 34 seconds. These factors were the robotic platform, surgical technique and the surgeon's skill. Even with the great differences, the general pattern showed that when the robots were used, the surgical team and the patient had a reduced radiation exposure, which was a major safety benefit (Li et al., 2020).

In addition, the systematic review from 2017 looked into the problem of learning curve in the case of robotic spine surgery. Nine different research works studied the impact of surgeon's experience on the time taken for surgery and the improvements in accuracy through successive cases. Registration failures, soft-tissue interference and lateral skiving of drill guides were the most common difficulties that were recognized. The results show that although robotic systems have excellent precision, their working at peak performance relies on the surgeon's familiarity and technical skill. Therefore, continuous training and refinement of the system are necessary to reduce errors and increase the clinical outcomes (Soomro et al., 2020).

3.4 Summary of Meta-Data Table

Table 1. Comparative Outcomes of Robotic-Assisted vs. Conventional/Freehand/Fluoroscopy-Guided Spine Instrumentation

Outcome	Robotic Assisted	Conventional / Freehand / Fluoro	Findings / Supporting Evidence
Screw breach / misplacement	Significantly fewer breaches in many analyses (e.g., OR = 0.54; OR = 2.61, 95% CI: 1.75–3.91, P < 0.0001)	Higher breach incidence and greater variability in placement accuracy	Robotic systems show superior accuracy and consistency in pedicle screw placement; AR slightly exceeds robotics in facet joint protection (Li et al., 2020; Naik et al., 2022; Riewruja et al., 2024; Cui et al., 2024).
Neurologic complications	Lower incidence; improved safety profiles due to higher screw trajectory precision	Higher complication rates linked to malposition and cortical breaches	Robotic guidance reduces neurologic risk and improves intraoperative confidence (Łajczak et al., 2024; Vadalà et al., 2020).
Blood loss	Generally lower mean difference (MD = −112.7 mL in one meta-analysis); minimal intraoperative trauma	Higher average intraoperative blood loss	Some analyses found no significant reduction, but consistent trend toward less bleeding (Li et al., 2020; Tarawneh et al., 2021).

continued on following page

Table 1. Continued

Outcome	Robotic Assisted	Conventional / Freehand / Fluoro	Findings / Supporting Evidence
Operative time	Longer operative and setup time (+43.6 min on average in scoliosis meta-analysis)	Shorter; established workflow	Longer time attributed to registration and learning curve; efficiency improves with experience (Cui et al., 2024; Soomro et al., 2020).
Hospital stays	Slightly shorter (−1.12 days on average); faster recovery in minimally invasive approaches	Comparable or slightly longer	Some meta-analyses show marginal benefit; effect may depend on case complexity (Li et al., 2020).
Radiation exposure / Fluoroscopy	Reduced exposure for surgical team and patient (fluoroscopy time 1.3–34 sec per screw)	Higher or variable depending on surgeon skill and imaging protocol	Robot-assisted and AR systems reduce cumulative radiation exposure, though data remain heterogeneous (Li et al., 2020; MacLean et al., 2024).
Safety (overall complication rate)	Comparable or slightly improved; fewer revision surgeries and screw-related reoperations	Similar or higher; dependent on experience and imaging accuracy	Robotic use enhances procedural reproducibility and safety margins; further long-term trials needed (Huang et al., 2021; Łajczak et al., 2024).
Learning curve / Training	Requires dedicated training; performance improves with surgeon experience	Familiar workflow; minimal adaptation needed	Robotic accuracy depends on user proficiency; errors due to registration failure and soft-tissue interference noted (Soomro et al., 2020).

3.5 Interpretation

The evidence indicates that robotic aid for spinal instrumentation has evolved to demonstrate real benefits for accuracy of screw placement and rates of breaches and neuromuscular complication for certain indications. Yet, improvements are not universal and depend on the specific surgical indication (degenerative, deformity, trauma), the robot platform, the experience of the surgeon, the workflow/institutional structure and patient anatomical configuration. Most importantly, many meta-analyses and reviews indicate that, although there was enhancement in accuracy, clinical outcomes (pain relief, function, fusion rate, time to revision) are less described and are the target of future studies.

4. REAL-WORLD APPLICATIONS

4.1 Indications and Use-Cases

Robotic spinal instrumentation has proven valuable in various surgical contexts. Examples of surgical indications include posterior lumbar and thoracolumbar pedicle screw fixation for degenerative diseases and spondylolisthesis, as well as MIS approaches for percutaneous pedicle screws. In addition, robotics has been applied in spinal deformity corrections such as scoliosis and kyphosis; as well as complex revision cases for established instrumentation or altered anatomy that made nerve root and pedicle screw placement difficult. While cervical spine applications are less established, early studies have documented the feasibility of robotics in these settings. For example, in segmental scoliosis instrumentation, the robotic placement of screws had clinically acceptable accuracy in comparison to freehand with an odds ratio of 2.61. Robotic instrumentation was more time-consuming but was documented as to accuracy and the postoperative assessment described in the PubMed meta-analysis of robotic pedicle screw placement accuracy and postoperative assessment of robotic pedicle screw placement.

4.2 Clinical Workflow Integration

The robotic system is integrated into the operating room (OR) workflow in a systematic way, with technology assisting the process throughout. This process generally begins with preoperative planning based on CT-based imaging or immediate intraoperative imaging using CT/O-arm for precise anatomic registration of the operation table patient. After the patient has been registered, the robotic arm or guidance platform is precisely positioned. This positioning process requires precise cooperation among the attending surgeon, the scrub nurse, the imaging personnel and the navigation or robotics technician. After completing the desired, the imaging verification is used to confirm the accuracy of the screw trajectories. Data is also recorded for quality assurance purposes in the surgical workflows and verifying the images trajectory positions. The introduction of robotics and surgical navigation technology afforded the surgeon with a greater level of security, especially related to procedures that were minimally invasive or smaller access operations as the need for tactile feedback was considerably less, and the potential for reoperations was reduced based on screw malposition from imaging trajectory verification.

4.3 Institutional Impact

Institutional adoption of robotic spine surgery involves both operational and strategic implications. Robotic platforms, intraoperative imaging systems, and navigation devices require substantial capital investment. In addition to these devices, training of both the operating room staff and the surgeons will experience a learning curve as they engage in comprehensive training, during which they may extend surgical time experiencing robots for the first time. Further, to maintain programming and infrastructure, the robotic systems will also require some maintenance. Despite these limitations, robotics offer a hospital marketing opportunity and clinical presence; robotics also offers a competitive advantage. In most cases, hospitals will introduce robotic-assisted implementation starting with relatively simple cases such as single-level lumbar fusions or other easy surgical indications before progressing into complex deformity and revision surgery cases based on experience in robotic use.

4.4 Challenges and Limitations

Even with technological progress, robotic spine instrumentation still encounters a number of workflow and technical challenges. One prominent issue is registration error, which occurs when the alignment of the patient's anatomy coordinates does not accurately correspond to the robotic guidance system. Issues with registration can limit the advantages of robotic assistance in spine instrumentation procedures and could lead to potential screw misalignment. This highlights an important flaw: the rigid precision of the surgical robot is in contradiction to the moving, living anatomy of the patient undergoing surgery on the surgical table. Including other errors - the calibration error with the system, motion of the intraoperative reference frame, and the difficult requirement to obtain imaging confirmation for each intraoperative decision made, is an indication of the need for improved registration techniques and system reliability, but more importantly, maintaining awareness intraoperatively to fulfill the potential of surgical robotics in spine instrumentation.

4.5 Current Applications for Robotics in Spine Surgery

Robotic-assisted spine surgery has significantly progressed, yet numerous practical barriers still exist. One main barrier is skiving, or soft-tissue interference, which occurs when the drill guide or robotic arm slips on the bony surface or is displaced by moving soft tissues. As the result of either of these occurrences, there can be a discrepancy between the planned screw trajectory and the actual screw trajectory. Robotic workflows also tend to be based on intraoperative imaging, often of high-quality (O-arm or cone-beam CT [CBCT]), which can contribute to both equipment burden, as well as avoidable radiation exposure when preoperative or between-shot images would have sufficed. Early clinical series indicate a longer operative time with robotic-assisted cases (scoliosis cases had an average additional 43 minutes), often associated with setup time, registration, and inefficiencies related to the workflow. Failure of the robotic system, including inaccurate registrations or robotic arm failures, may result in conversion back to traditional techniques to avoid complications, and of course, this adds time to the surgical case. While some studies indicate reduced radiation exposure for surgeon and the operating team and associated staff, thus far, the findings have been variable and are dependent on imaging protocols and surgical approach.

4.6 Economic and Cost-Effectiveness Issues

The economic viability of robotic spine surgery continues to be a significant worry. Robotic systems can have a high entry price point for hardware and for imaging or navigation infrastructure components which can be an acute financial burden for most smaller centers. Although enhanced screw placement accuracy has been shown, there is still insufficient evidence to show a link between robotic use and improved long-term outcomes such as fusion rates, revision attempts, or overall savings. One published systematic review stated that there was no conclusive advantage to robotic spinal fusion over freehand spinal fusion with respect to clinical outcomes. In addition, the hidden costs of maintenance of the equipment, consumable items such as sterile drapes and surgical guides, and time spent training the surgeon and operating room personnel complicate the cost-benefit calculus. For low-volume or resource-limited hospitals, this expense can only be justified by having quality operating room personnel and/or demand for surgical procedures that are often complex.

4.7 Evidence Gaps and Clinical Outcomes

The majority of the current research on robotic spine surgery has focused on technical accuracy metrics (e.g. accuracy of screw placement or rates of breach) and lacks long-term clinical metrics (e.g. rates of fusion, hardware failure, patient-reported satisfaction, cost-utility). *A critical gap persists between technical success and patient benefit. We meticulously measure the precision of the screw's journey but remain uncertain of its final destination: improved long-term patient well-being.* Furthermore, there is a considerable level of heterogeneity across the entirety of the research base, including robotic platform, surgical experience, definitions of accuracy, or surgical indications, that makes it difficult to compare to other studies. There are also concerns regarding publication bias, as some meta-analyses indicate potential bias in up to 60% of Tirobot studies and up to 30% of Spine Assist publications. Only a limited number of high-quality randomized controlled trials (RCT) have reported either long-term follow-up or some form of cost-effectiveness analysis, indicating the need for higher levels of quality and more extensive research to truly understand the value of robotic assisted spine surgery and if it can sustain itself in the future.

4.8 Adoption, Training, and Human Factors

The incorporation of robotics into spine surgery concludes a complete paradigm shift in the surgical workflow which requires a paradigm shift from members of the surgical team. In addition to the technical cost, the psychological cost of the swing in technology makes some surgeons feel de-skilled. Training will need to establish a collaborative mindset in addition to the technical skills. The surgeon will need to transition from the traditional free-hand tactile technique to a method of robot-assisted planning and positioning. In addition to the surgeon, the dynamics of the operating room team will be different, requiring new roles like a robotic technician, and cooperation in acquiring imaging, positioning the robot-guided instrumentation, and verifying position of the robot-guided instrumentation. There are certainly challenges to implementation due to resistance to change, perceived complexities of the procedure, and lengthening case times, but these should not impede widespread utilization and acceptance. Successful implementation will require structured training programs and processes for credentialing the surgeon; and the surgical team needs to be comfortable with having a plan, should the system not operate as planned, including a conversion to a manual technique. Furthermore, the interface between the human and the robots will continue to develop, as the ergonomics of the robotic systems must also evolve to allow the surgeon to still maintain control of the robot, while the robot provides precision and autonomy.

4.9 Emerging and Future Challenges

The future of robotic spine surgery will benefit from utilizing advanced technologies, such as artificial intelligence (AI) and machine learning, so profound improvements could be achieved in preoperative modeling, adaptable intraoperative procedure, and the accuracy of screw placement prediction. New technologies, such as augmentative reality (AR) and mixed reality (MR) technologies, may be able to surpass current state-of-the-art navigation and robotic systems due to recent meta-analyses suggesting these technologies to be up to 85% accurate within surgical navigation and patient interbody alignment. However, the current pursuit of fully automated robots to independently drill or insert screws remains in the experimental phase and has many regulatory, safety, and ethical issues that would come into consideration. In order for robotics to be adopted clinically, costs must be reduced and ways to use robots developed to be more accessible. The problem is even worse in low- and middle-income areas. Exploring wider research areas and expanding the scope of robots to do more than pedicle screw placement for interbody fusions, deformity correction, and osteotomies. Additionally, it is important to create standard metrics for performance, standard definitions for complication, and standardized reporting method for cost-effective reporting to enhance inter-study comparisons and meta-analysis, in the many evolving paradigms.

5. CASE VOLUME AND CASE MIX

Prior to proceeding with instrumentation in robotics, a few general recommendations for a surgical center or spine surgical group are to look closely at their case volume and case complexity. If the center has exceptionally large case volume, especially to make "complex deformity corrections or revisions," this can mitigate the financial investment in robotics and subsequent ability to recoup financial obligations for the surgical team, because of the precision, accuracy and consistency that the robot provides – especially when it concerns spine surgery.

5.1 Infrastructure Readiness

When doing robotic spine surgery, there is a need for a strong supportive infrastructure. This is especially true for intra-operative 3D imaging systems such as O-arm or cone-beam CT (CBCT) and for having a navigation system that one can depend on. In addition, institutions must have trained technicians and/or biomedical engineers to assist with setup, calibration and troubleshooting of the system during the surgical case.

5.2 Surgeon and Team Training

For patient safety and efficiency, robotic-assisted spine surgery requires some structured education for the surgeon and surgical team. Surgeons and surgical teams need to complete a structured educational program that includes simulation, supervised cases, and proctored cases by a busy, advanced robotic surgeon. Instructional early cases under supervision and realistic expectations for the learning curve and early increased operative setup time is still supported.

5.3 Workflow Optimization

The process of streamlining a workflow is critical to reducing operative time and aiding in standardization across cases. Standardization should focus on components of the workflow that will impact items related to preoperative planning, patient registration, positioning of the robotic arm and verification imaging. An effective workflow will result in an increased degree of efficiency, less intra-operative variability and improved reliability of the integration of robotic surgery into the operating room.

5.4 Data Collection and Audit

The ongoing and continuous collection and auditing of data is essential if we want to help understand and justify the use of robotics. Hospitals or institutions will want to track important outcomes metrics, such as accuracy of screw placement and breach rate, operative time, complications, radiation metrics, cost metrics, and revision rate. In addition to improving your surgical protocols, the audits will allow you to trace the trajectory of improvements.

5.5 Cost-Effectiveness Modelling

In order to prepare for a broad deployment, institutions need to examine the cost-effectiveness of the policy. This is assessing cost per case, and possible savings from revision surgery or liability due to malpositioned screws, and surgical throughput. Decision-makers can use financial modeling to confirm the value of this investment relates to institutional priorities and is sustainable over the long term.

5.6 Patient Selection

During the early phase of deployment, robotic spine surgery may best be suited for patients to whom screw placement accuracy would be advantageous. These cases may include a spinal deformity, osteoporotic bone, and/or revision surgery. The intention of selective use, at least during the early phase, would be to allow the teams the experience and expertise for or outcomes that are best, in case of complications or heightened situational stress.

5.7 Contingency Planning

Despite advancements in technology, a system error or failure can occur during surgery. Therefore, teams should include contingency plans to promote continuity of safe care and surgical process. Surgeons and the operating room team must recognize that if the robotic registration or navigation fails, they can revert to their practice patterns of freehand or fluoroscopic guided placement of screws to ensure continued surgical advancement and avoid operating room delays.

5.8 Role of the Medical Education Department

The Division of Medical Education is central to the evaluation, development, and continuous enhancement of training in robotic spine surgery. The Division of Medical Education is invested in the curricular infusion of robotic spine surgery education and multiple forms of simulation-based education, interprofessional education, and on-going competency assessments as it applies to robotic-assisted surgery technologies. In creating the trainings, it must cover the gap between theory and practice, and include aspects of crisis and teamwork, as well as provide a safe environment to learn about real-life complications.

The departments of medical education in neurosurgery and orthopedics have begun to work collaboratively to plan systematic approaches, in which components of a theoretical basis and technical skills learning together form the medicinal aspect. The simulation and skills laboratory, as well as practice areas featuring virtual reality and robotic training have permitted the opportunity to have staff, the doctors, the residents and operating room staff, to engage in task simulation before they take on the duty and responsibility of patient care. Educational approaches will shorten the learning curve, reduce the error count in surgery, and better teamwork in practice. The Medical Education Division keeps track of credential and certification documentation, and ensures the organizations maintain compliance with the accreditation standards. In addition, the Division provides professional development for staff through workshops and continuing medical education (CME), and through interdisciplinary grand rounds covering the case-based experiences, the innovations, and the challenges of robotic surgery. Medical educational units at research-intensive institutions act as facilitators of dissemination for academic initiatives encompassing areas such as the fidelity of simulation, the effectiveness of training, and the impact of robotic instruction on patient safety and performance among others. The Medical Education Division promotes a culture of continuous learning and reflection, serving as a conduit between evolving surgical technology, and safe, evidence-based clinical practice.

6. FUTURE DIRECTIONS AND RESEARCH PRIORITIES

The previously referenced scope in a number of aspects warrants a high degree of focus regarding clinical trials and technology advancement for spinal surgery with robots. Practical randomized controlled trials (RCTs) with long follow-up that employ direct comparative methods between robotic compared to traditional techniques is critical and would facilitate a direct comparison of outcomes such as fusion rates, revision surgery rates, patient-reported outcomes measures (PROM), and quality-adjusted life years (QALY) ultimately to allow for cost-utility analysis. Additionally, areas that would warrant the use of a standardized reporting framework may include harmonized definitions around accuracy (Gertzbein-Robbins classification), definitions of screw breach, definitions of radiation dose, and definitions of operative time across the trials. Studies that are comparative among platforms are also very important. They will include direct comparisons between robotic systems (for example, Mazor X, TiRobot, ROSA) and would provide an overall synthesis through Network meta-analyses to get best in class platform; some pilot projects have started on this topic. Furthermore, the community that is integrating navigation, AR/VR technologies with robotic systems, is now seen as the one that guarantees the most efficient surgical workflow and the best surgical outcomes; for instance, combining robotic guidance with AR for visualization. The systemization and support of decisions should be driven by automation in the future with a strong focus on AI robotic-assisted surgical planning, using the patient-specific anatomy and bone quality to optimize screw trajectories, along with intraoperative force sensing and monitoring with a view towards possible future autonomous robotic insertion under human oversight without pitfalls. Additional cost reduction strategies are needed to democratize access by focusing on volume/build modular, mobile, affordable robotic systems to even effectively serve (low) resource settings and also extending to procedures that address the gap of surgeon training models scalable to build competence. Another significant area for robotics development is expanded use in minimally invasive techniques and a range of devices such as extreme lateral interbody fusion, anterior spine instrumentation, cervical spine devices, and possibly multi-rod instrumentation for deformity correction. It would still require additional research that quantifies the (significance of) radiations dose reductions to surgeons, staff, and patients and/or safer working environment and practice to influence those research trajectories when a mechanical system has been introduced. The future lies in intelligent systems that augment the surgeon. These "cognitive" partners will offer predictive warnings and adaptive planning, transforming the robot from a tool into a collaborative assistant. And lastly, further understanding of the learning curve is needed to determine goal of further studies towards quantifying the number of cases needed to reach competence in improved accuracy, reduced intra-op workflow, or outcomes stratified by (multiple levels) of prior expertise and surgical experience for the surgeon.

7. CONCLUSION

The use of surgical robotics for spine instrumentation represents a major advance in spinal surgery. Meta-analyses and systematic reviews provide reasonable evidence of improved accuracy in screw placement, lower rates of breach and neurologic complications, and possibly less blood loss and decreased length of stay in some populations. However, we have not yet transitioned those possible benefits into improved long-term patient-centered outcomes, cost-effectiveness, and widespread application. There are components critical to a successful implementation, including appropriate institutional planning, education, training and credentialing of surgeons and teams, workflow adaptation, and performance criterion monitoring. Future studies should continue to investigate long-term outcomes, comparative effectiveness of platforms, integration with new technology (e.g., navigation, augmented reality, artificial intelligence), economics, and application of robotic systems across a variety of health-care systems. For health-care systems and individual practitioners considering adoption, utilizing the robotic platform during high-complexity cases (e.g., deformity, revision surgery) could offer the most promise; systematic use of the robotic system for all cases, including routine and simple cases, should be assessed for relative cost and logistical burden. In the end, when robotics, navigation, and AI come together, we might just be ready for a new generation of spine implants characterized by increased precision, safety, and efficiency — however, it is still our duty to be cautious and choose based on evidence. The very flourishing of surgical robots is not the result of their high-tech development but rather our ability to apply that technology together with the patient's needs in mind.

REFERENCES

Anokwute, M. C., Obeng-Gyasi, B., Chinthala, A. S., Savage, J., & Mao, G. (2025). Robotic Spine Fusion Bridges the Surgeon Learning Gap: A 5-Year Analysis of Screw Placement Accuracy and Efficiency Between Experienced and Inexperienced Surgeons. *World Neurosurgery: X*, •••, 100513.

Cui, W., Liu, X., Zhao, Z., Feng, Z., & Meng, X. (2024). Accuracy and postoperative assessment of robot-assisted placement of pedicle screws during scoliosis surgery compared with conventional freehand technique: A systematic review and meta-analysis. *Journal of Orthopaedic Surgery and Research*, *19*(1), 365. PMID: 38902785

Fatima, N., Massaad, E., Hadzipasic, M., Shankar, G. M., & Shin, J. H. (2021). Safety and accuracy of robot-assisted placement of pedicle screws compared to conventional free-hand technique: A systematic review and meta-analysis. *The Spine Journal*, *21*(2), 181–192. PMID: 32976997

Galieri, G., Orlando, V., Altieri, R., Barbarisi, M., Olivi, A., Sabatino, G., & La Rocca, G. (2025). Current Trends and Future Directions in Lumbar Spine Surgery: A Review of Emerging Techniques and Evolving Management Paradigms. *Journal of Clinical Medicine*, *14*(10), 3390. PMID: 40429385

Gautam, D., Vivekanandan, S., & Mazur, M. D. (2025). Robotic spine surgery: Systematic review of common error types and best practices. *Operative Neurosurgery (Hagerstown, Md.)*, *28*(3), 295–302. PMID: 39037253

Hammond, J., & Priola, S. (2025). Advancements in robotic-assisted spine surgery: A literature review and technology comparison. *Interdisciplinary Neurosurgery : Advanced Techniques and Case Management*, •••, 102056.

Hammond, J., & Priola, S. (2025). Advancements in robotic-assisted spine surgery: A literature review and technology comparison. *Interdisciplinary Neurosurgery : Advanced Techniques and Case Management*, •••, 102056.

Huang, M., Tetreault, T. A., Vaishnav, A., York, P. J., & Staub, B. N. (2021). The current state of navigation in robotic spine surgery. *Annals of Translational Medicine*, *9*(1), 86. PMID: 33553379

Łajczak, P., Żerdziński, K., Jóźwik, K., Laskowski, M., & Dymek, M. (2024). Enhancing precision and safety in spinal surgery: A comprehensive review of robotic assistance technologies. *World Neurosurgery*, *191*, 109–116. PMID: 39151699

Li, H. M., Zhang, R. J., & Shen, C. L. (2020). Accuracy of pedicle screw placement and clinical outcomes of robot-assisted technique versus conventional freehand technique in spine surgery from nine randomized controlled trials: A meta-analysis. *Spine*, *45*(2), E111–E119. PMID: 31404053

Li, J., Fang, Y., Jin, Z., Wang, Y., & Yu, M. (2020). The impact of robot-assisted spine surgeries on clinical outcomes: A systemic review and meta-analysis. *International Journal of Medical Robotics and Computer Assisted Surgery*, *16*(6), 1–14. PMID: 32725898

Li, T., Yan, J., Li, J., Shang, Y., & Tang, X. (2025). Robot-assisted technique versus freehand technique for spine surgery: An umbrella review. *Annals of Medicine*, *57*(1), 2523564. PMID: 40631354

Liu, Z., Huang, J., Zhang, H., Zhang, S., Dai, H., Jiang, Y., & Shan, Z. (2025). The application of robotic and artificial intelligence technologies in spinal surgery: A review focused on prospects in remote areas of China. *Journal of Robotic Surgery*, *19*(1), 1–17. PMID: 40940589

MacLean, L., Hersh, A. M., Bhimreddy, M., Jiang, K., Davidar, A. D., Weber-Levine, C., ... & Theodore, N. (2024). Comparison of accuracy, revision, and perioperative outcomes in robot-assisted spine surgeries: systematic review and meta-analysis. *Journal of Neurosurgery: Spine, 1*(aop), 1-13.

Malham, G. M., Wells-Quinn, T. A., Nowitzke, A. M., Mobbs, R. J., & Sekhon, L. H. (2024). Challenges in contemporary spinal robotics: Encouraging spine surgeons to drive transformative changes in the development of future robotic platforms. *Journal of Spine Surgery*, *10*(3), 540. PMID: 39399084

Naik, A., Smith, A. D., Shaffer, A., Krist, D. T., Moawad, C. M., MacInnis, B. R., & Arnold, P. M. (2022). Evaluating robotic pedicle screw placement against conventional modalities: A systematic review and network meta-analysis. *Neurosurgical Focus*, *52*(1), E10. PMID: 34973681

Riewruja, K., Tanasansomboon, T., Yingsakmongkol, W., Kotheeranurak, V., Limthongkul, W., Chokesuwattanaskul, R., & Singhatanadgige, W. (2024). A Network Meta-Analysis Comparing the Efficacy and Safety of Pedicle Screw Placement Techniques Using Intraoperative Conventional, Navigation, Robot-Assisted, and Augmented Reality Guiding Systems. *The International Journal of Spine Surgery*, *18*(5), 551–570. PMID: 39079746

Samprón, N., Lafuente, J., Presa-Alonso, J., Ivanov, M., Hartl, R., & Ringel, F. (2025). Advancing spine surgery: Evaluating the potential for full robotic automation. *Brain & Spine*, •••, 104232. PMID: 40191588

Schneider, D., Brown, E. D., Elsamadicy, A. A., Sciubba, D. M., & Lo, S. F. L. (2025). The Hidden Cost of Robotic Spine Surgery: Real-World Adverse Events Cause 58-Minute Delays and Undermine Economic Viability. *The Spine Journal*.

Schneider, D., Brown, E. D., Elsamadicy, A. A., Sciubba, D. M., & Lo, S. F. L. (2025). The Hidden Cost of Robotic Spine Surgery: Real-World Adverse Events Cause 58-Minute Delays and Undermine Economic Viability. *The Spine Journal*.

Soomro, N. A., Hashimoto, D. A., Porteous, A. J., Ridley, C. J. A., Marsh, W. J., Ditto, R., & Roy, S. (2020). Systematic review of learning curves in robot-assisted surgery. *BJS Open*, *4*(1), 27–44. PMID: 32011823

Sridhar, A. N., Briggs, T. P., Kelly, J. D., & Nathan, S. (2017). Training in robotic surgery—An overview. *Current Urology Reports*, *18*(8), 58. PMID: 28647793

Sun, W. X., Huang, W. Q., Li, H. Y., Wang, H. S., Guo, S. L., Dong, J., & Lin, Y. P. (2023). Clinical efficacy of robotic spine surgery: An updated systematic review of 20 randomized controlled trials. *EFORT Open Reviews*, *8*(11), 841–853. PMID: 37909700

Sun, W. X., Huang, W. Q., Li, H. Y., Wang, H. S., Guo, S. L., Dong, J., & Lin, Y. P. (2023). Clinical efficacy of robotic spine surgery: An updated systematic review of 20 randomized controlled trials. *EFORT Open Reviews*, *8*(11), 841–853. PMID: 37909700

Susskind, R. (2025). *How to Think about AI: A Guide for the Perplexed*. Oxford University Press.

Tarawneh, A. M., & Salem, K. M. (2021). A systematic review and meta-analysis of randomized controlled trials comparing the accuracy and clinical outcome of pedicle screw placement using robot-assisted technology and conventional freehand technique. *Global Spine Journal*, *11*(4), 575–586. PMID: 32677515

Vadalà, G., De Salvatore, S., Ambrosio, L., Russo, F., Papalia, R., & Denaro, V. (2020). Robotic spine surgery and augmented reality systems: A state of the art. *Neurospine*, *17*(1), 88. PMID: 32252158

Wang, Y., Xiao, Y., Wang, J., Rexiti, P., & Wang, Y. (2025). Spine-specific robots may offer superior screw placement accuracy in spinal surgery procedures. A systematic review and network and proportional meta-analysis. *Journal of Orthopaedic Surgery and Research*, *20*(1), 1–23. PMID: 41137102

Chapter 8
Data-Driven Prediction of Brain Stroke Risk Using Machine Learning Techniques on Healthcare

Muhammad Bilal Ashraf
https://orcid.org/0000-0002-8079-3535
Freie Universiat Berlin, Germany

ABSTRACT

A brain stroke is a very serious health issue that is responsible for about 10% of death cases all over the world (nearly 6 million people) in 2019, and it is one of the top 10 causes of death and long-term disability in many countries. The medical community tries to turn this around by focusing on early diagnosis and treatment. Usually, other methods may not be available in developing regions where diagnosis and treatment are done using primitive tools. This project aims to employ the ever-increasing electronic health records together with data science to develop a predictive model that will detect high-risk individuals over stroke based on their health and lifestyle factors. The research is based on the Brain Stroke Dataset from Kaggle, which contains 4981 records with 11 attributes, including age, hypertension, heart disease, and smoking habits as the most important ones.

DOI: 10.4018/979-8-3373-6234-2.ch008

1. INTRODUCTION

A brain stroke is an event that results in the death of brain tissue as a consequence of the interruption of blood flow to the brain. There are two primary categories of strokes: ischemic and hemorrhagic; the latter being the less common form. An ischemic stroke can also be referred to as a cerebral infarction, and it occurs when one of the arteries supplying the brain is obstructed, and consequently, less blood reaches the brain, which eventually injures the brain tissues. In contrast, a hemorrhagic stroke is characterized by bleeding in the brain caused by a ruptured blood vessel. Strokes are the leading cause of death worldwide and are also responsible for a lot of disabilities and difficulties that affect not only the patients but also the health systems globally (Salleh et al., 2021; WHO, 2024).

Stroke risk factors are composed of both modifiable and non-modifiable versions. High blood pressure is the number one modifiable risk factor, and it is followed by diabetes, smoking, obesity, and high levels of cholesterol. On the other hand, the non-modifiable factors like age, gender, race, and heredity are naturally beyond control. The older a person gets, the higher the chance of a stroke occurring, and some population groups are more vulnerable to strokes. And even in some low-income countries, the stroke incidence rate is significantly high due to poor working conditions and the poverty level (Jain, 2019; Boehme et al., 2017).

Preventive measures are essential in reducing the risk of brain strokes. Among them, the most effective ways to lower the risk of stroke are eating a healthy diet and exercising regularly. Those who are diagnosed with high blood pressure, diabetes, or high cholesterol have the option of significantly lowering their risk of stroke by taking doctor-recommended medications, among other methods. In certain circumstances, the medical community may intervene to perform carotid endarterectomy or stenting to reduce the risk of brain strokes even more. It is very important that people who are at risk of stroke are informed and helped to prioritize early detection, managing risk factors, and adopting a lifestyle of healthy habits to control the occurrence of brain strokes (Howard & Mcdonnell, 2015). The digitalization of health records and the ongoing advancements in data science have made it possible to perform an analysis of large health datasets, which is a very promising way for the early prediction of brain stroke risk. The Brain Stroke Dataset, which is available on Kaggle and comprises health and demographic data of more than 4,981 people, is a great resource for the identification of important factors related to stroke risk using data-driven approaches. This project is going to apply the techniques of data science to determine the risk of stroke based on the health data. By looking at the Stroke Prediction Dataset present on Kaggle, this initiative wants to reveal the patterns and associations that can help predict the likelihood of a stroke occurring and understanding the risks associated with strokes (Raju, 2024).

2. LITERATURE REVIEW

The primary objective of this project is to create a model that utilizes data as its principal resource and an individual's health profile as its foundation to forecast the probability of that individual experiencing a stroke. Given the severity of strokes, which can lead to death, the prompt identification of individuals at high risk would significantly enhance their chances of recovery if appropriate actions were taken swiftly. Consequently, the "Healthcare Dataset for Stroke Prediction" has been chosen to explore and assess the strength of the correlation between stroke risk and various factors such as age, heart disease, hypertension, BMI, blood sugar levels, different occupations, along with other demographic and health-related variables.

Additionally, the project seeks to promote wellness through the application of predictive analytics, enabling preventive measures in health risk areas to be implemented effectively. A dataset that has been reviewed preliminarily will be subjected to basic exploratory analysis that will unearth its main traits. The first step is to assess the features with the most significant influence on the study outcome. The notable features are age, BMI and glucose level. We also look at the distribution of those features, notice if there are any missing values, and validate the up-to-date statistics by means of checking their responsiveness (mean, median, and range) to the main components. However, in addition to the visual inspection of features and their relationships to stroke outcomes, the application of correlation analysis will also point out the early trends (Amann, 2022).

Next, we move on to the data preprocessing phase that comprises all cleansing and preparation tasks that are necessary for machine learning to be effective. Processing of the data in this case involves the handling of the categorical variables of fleet gender and work type, and numeric values adjustment, if necessary. At this stage, the data must be free of bias and error to such an extent that they would not detract from the model's prediction accuracy (Singh et al., 2025).

Poor health conditions were among the main parameters in the classification process, and through these steps, the likelihood of a stroke was predicted by means of logistic regression. Random Forest Classifier was further involved in setting the significance of the different features in stroke prediction, besides providing the highest predictive accuracy, and identifying the main factors affecting stroke risk. The aforementioned classifier was also assisted by a Decision Tree Classifier which made a user-friendly model through rules that, in turn, would help form unambiguous decisions. The model's aim is to offer a simple and clear visual that not only depicts the reasoning behind the feature values that lead to the classification of a certain case as stroke or non-stroke but also links the two. In addition, Support Vector Machines (SVM) were deployed to obtain the intricate and non-linear decision boundaries (Bhuria and Sudheer, 2025). The objective of the model is to distinguish between stroke and non-stroke cases by a soft margin while simultaneously depicting the effect of two crucial features in the classification. The K-Means Clustering technique was combined with PCA (Principal Component Analysis) to reduce the feature size and find the inherent data groups, all this without providing any labels for the data. The aim of this model is to disclose specific patient subgroups, defined by their health condition, that are predisposed to stroke and thus signal the possibility of sub-categorization in the overall population. In addition to that, through linear regression, the study tried to investigate the health factors and their influence on the outcomes (Ahmed et al., 2024).

The model's goal is to explore the connection between the patient's age and his BMI, which in turn, will provide an idea of how age may influence the body mass index of patients with stroke. The use of these methods enabled the research to examine more profoundly the elements that could increase stroke risk and consequently, the early detection of individuals in high-risk groups and better health policies (Alanazi et al., 2025; Chahine et al., 2023) would be the result.

During the machine learning process, we carry out at the end of the steps a model validation exercise which exercises the accuracy of the developed models. This process involves partitioning the data into training and testing sets, followed by the application of cross-validation, along with evaluation using various data-driven metrics. In classification tasks, we utilize confusion matrices to calculate accuracy, precision, recall, and F1-score. For clustering purposes, we evaluate the quality of the clusters by using the Silhouette Score, Davies-Bouldin Index, and Calinski-Harabasz Index (Thakre et al., 2025; Nayak and Gupta, 2024). In regression analysis, the Mean Squared Error (MSE) and R^2 score are employed as the primary metrics to assess the model's performance. All these steps make sure that our models are not only accurate and reliable but also safe for medical use. Validation of models has been one of the aspects of our clear and simple step-by-step process, which started from basic statistics and went through the whole process of model validation. The study shows that data application can not only provide a better understanding of stroke risks but also a quicker response in health care (Lee et al., 2024).

3. DESCRIPTION OF DATA SET

The dataset includes health records of 4,981 people which were gathered to analyze and predict stroke occurrences. It is organized in such a way that relationships between individuals, demographic factors, and health-related variables (like medical conditions and health behaviors) can be investigated. This data is of great importance for healthcare analytics and machine learning aimed at early detection and prevention, as shown in Figure 1.

Figure 1. first 20 records of the brain_stroke_dataset

	A	B	C	D	E	F	G	H	I	J	K
1	gender	age	hypertension	heart_disease	ever_married	work_type	Residence_type	avg_glucose_level	bmi	smoking_status	stroke
2	Male	67	0	1	Yes	Private	Urban	228.69	36.6	formerly smoked	1
3	Male	80	0	1	Yes	Private	Rural	105.92	32.5	never smoked	1
4	Female	49	0	0	Yes	Private	Urban	171.23	34.4	smokes	1
5	Female	79	1	0	Yes	Self-emplc	Rural	174.12	24	never smoked	1
6	Male	81	0	0	Yes	Private	Urban	186.21	29	formerly smoked	1
7	Male	74	1	1	Yes	Private	Rural	70.09	27.4	never smoked	1
8	Female	69	0	0	No	Private	Urban	94.39	22.8	never smoked	1
9	Female	78	0	0	Yes	Private	Urban	58.57	24.2	Unknown	1
10	Female	81	1	0	Yes	Private	Rural	80.43	29.7	never smoked	1
11	Female	61	0	1	Yes	Govt_job	Rural	120.46	36.8	smokes	1
12	Female	54	0	0	Yes	Private	Urban	104.51	27.3	smokes	1
13	Female	79	0	1	Yes	Private	Urban	214.09	28.2	never smoked	1
14	Female	50	1	0	Yes	Self-emplc	Rural	167.41	30.9	never smoked	1
15	Male	64	0	1	Yes	Private	Urban	191.61	37.5	smokes	1
16	Male	75	1	0	Yes	Private	Urban	221.29	25.8	smokes	1
17	Female	60	0	0	No	Private	Urban	89.22	37.8	never smoked	1
18	Female	71	0	0	Yes	Govt_job	Rural	193.94	22.4	smokes	1
19	Female	52	1	0	Yes	Self-emplc	Urban	233.29	48.9	never smoked	1
20	Female	79	0	0	Yes	Self-emplc	Urban	228.7	26.6	never smoked	1

The dataset consists of 11 variables, each of which provides information about a particular aspect of a person's profile.

The aspects mentioned are classified into the following three groups:

1. Demographic Features: Individuals' demographic information is included in this category such as age, gender, marital status, employment type, and place of residence. These factors are considered to be the social and environmental determinants of health.
2. Health Features: This category consists of the variables that describe clinical and biometric data, among them, body mass index (BMI), average blood glucose level, and the presence of hypertension and heart disease. The health-related variables might help to assess a person's medical condition together with the risks connected to it.
3. Lifestyle Features: The category focuses on personal health habits, especially smoking status, which is a major risk factor for many chronic diseases, including stroke.

The stroke variable, which shows whether a person has had a stroke before (0 = No, 1 = Yes), is also one of the key endpoints that interest researchers in the area of modeling and statistical analysis, as it can be seen in Tables 1, 2, and 3.

Table 1. Demographic Features

Column Name	Data Type	Description	Example Values
gender	Categorical	Biological sex of the individual.	Male, Female
age	Float	Age of the individual in years.	67,80, 0.88
ever_married	Categorical	Whether the person has ever been married.	Yes, No
work_type	Categorical	Type of employment.	Private, Self-employed, Govt_job, children, Never_worked
residence_type	Categorical	Type of residence area.	Urban, Rural

Table 2. Health Features

Column Name	Data Type	Description	Example Values
hypertension	Integer	Indicates whether the person has high blood pressure.	0 = No, 1 = Yes
heart_disease	Integer	Indicates whether the person has any heart disease.	0 = No, 1 = Yes
avg_glucose_level	Float	Average blood glucose level (mg/dL).	228.69, 105.92
bmi	Float	Body Mass Index; missing in some records.	36.6, 32.5
stroke	Integer	Indicates whether the individual has experienced a stroke.	= No, 1 = Yes

Table 3. Lifestyle Features

Column Name	Data Type	Description	Example Values
smoking_status	Categorical	Smoking behavior of the individual	never smoked, smokes, formerly smoked, Unknown

5. METHODOLOGY

The work was done by conducting a strict and multi-faceted data science workflow which included data gathering, thorough cleaning and preprocessing, explorative data analysis (EDA), predictive modeling (classification), explorative clustering, and linear regression analysis.

5.1 Data Acquisition and Exploratory Data Analysis (EDA)

The identifier of the dataset was brain_stroke.csv, and it was the analyst's main focus, which was loaded through the conventional libraries of Python like pandas, NumPy, matplotlib, and scikit-learn. The data was frozen first by the shape of the Data Frame, the head, the tail, the info summary (info()), the descriptive statistics (describe()), counting missing values and duplicates. The exploratory analysis Rendered the first insights into the data structure. The insights consisted of calculating the range, skewness, and kurtosis of the numeric features, and, on top of that, determining the correlation of each numeric feature with the target variable, stroke. Some of the main visualizations made during EDA were: a histogram that depicts the Age distribution (with Kernel Density Estimate (KDE)) and a bar plot showing stroke frequency by work_type, a scatter graph juxtaposing Age and avg_glucose_level (with a fitted regression line), a boxplot that tells about BMI distribution split by stroke status, a pie chart that indicates gender distribution among stroke patients, and a line plot that presents the count of hypertensive and heart disease cases among smokers and non-smokers.

5.2 Data Preprocessing and Feature Engineering

The data cleaning consisted of the elimination of discrepancies and the preparation of features for the modeling. Missing values and duplicates were detected, and their counts were also provided. The standardization of string features was done on the following steps: the smoking_status column was replaced with underscores for all the whitespaces, and the terms work_type and smoking_status were written in uppercase letters to ensure uniformity. The column names such as Residence_type were also changed for similarity.

5.3 Outlier Mitigation and Transformation

The outlier detection in the age, avg_glucose_level, and bmi numerical columns were done by using the Interquartile Range (IQR) method, and the counts were printed prior to the transformation. To correct the skewness and reduce the influence of outliers, the Yeo-Johnson power transformation was performed on avg_glucose_level and bmi, which created the new columns glucose_yeojohnson and bmi_yeojohnson. The Yeo-Johnson transformation was chosen since it can handle zero or negative values without special treatment. Outlier counts were redone on the transformed variables to verify the reduction of extreme values. Even though the winsorize function was brought in, it was never utilized for the purpose of capping extreme values.

5.4 Encoding

Categorical variables such as gender, work_type, residence_type, and smoking_status were transformed into integers by means of the LabelEncoder. These encoders were preserved for possible inverse transformations. The binary feature ever_married was explicitly assigned to 0 and 1. After the transformation and encoding, the original non-transformed columns of avg_glucose_level and bmi were removed. The last preprocessed data was kept for reproducibility. Correlation heatmap was used to examine multicollinearity and relationships between features.

5.5 Modeling Strategy and Algorithms

The dataset after cleaning was split into training and test sets with the help of the train_test_split function. Because of the nature of stroke data, several strategies were applied: stratify=y was used during the splitting to keep the class proportions and class_weight='balanced' was applied in all classification models to avoid the bias towards the majority class was done explicitly.

5.6 Classification Models

The training and evaluation of four main classification algorithms

1. **Logistic Regression:** It was trained with parameters max_iter=1000 and class_weight='balanced'. The model coefficients were obtained and plotted to determine the influence of features on log-odds of stroke. Stacked histograms were used to visualize the predicted probabilities and to show the discrimination between stroke and non-stroke classes.
2. **Decision Tree:** The model was trained with the same class_weight='balanced' and limited max_depth=3 to preserve the interpreting capability of the model. Feature importances were visualized through plotting, and decision rules were viewed using plot_tree.
3. **Random Forest:** The model was trained with n_estimators=100 and max_depth=5, in addition class_weight='balanced' was also used. The feature importances of 10 best ones from the ensemble model were displayed through plotting.

4. **Support Vector Machine (SVM):** Use of RBF kernel with class_weight='balanced' was made. The complete model was trained on the entire features set. Besides, one instance dealing with age versus glucose_yeojohnson was scaled using StandardScaler and presented to show the decision boundary in a 2D space

5.7 Exploratory Techniques

In addition to predictive classification, the methodology also included two exploratory techniques:

1. Clustering (KMeans): PCA was utilized first to diminish the feature space to two components where noise and collinearity were greatly mitigated. KMeans was applied with K values varying from 2 to 7. The best cluster count (K=3) was determined from the silhouette scores. The final cluster summary presented the mean feature values per cluster and the number of members in each cluster.
2. Linear Regression: The experimental linear model took the age as input and predicted the output value of bmi_yeojohnson.

5.8 Validation and Evaluation

The current research aims to create a deep learning model that employs Convolutional Neural Networks (CNNs) to classify MRI brain images using the publicly available Brain Tumor MRI Dataset, provided by Masoud Nickparvar via Kaggle. This dataset comprises four categories: glioma, meningioma, pituitary tumor, and the absence of a tumor (Chetlapalli et al., 2018). The primary objective is to train a CNN model capable of accurately distinguishing between these categories, thereby assisting in clinical decision-making and improving diagnostic efficacy.

6. RESULT

This part explains the results of exploratory data analysis (EDA), predictive classification modeling, and the application of unsupervised learning methods on the dataset containing stroke risk.

6.1 Data Overview and Exploratory Analysis Findings

During exploratory analysis, the data characteristics and their distribution were observed. The numerical features that had the heaviest tails or were skewed include avg_glucose_level and bmi. The Interquartile Range (IQR) method for outlier detection brought up 602 outliers for avg_glucose_level and 43 for BMI.

6.2 Demographic and Health Trends

1. **Age Distribution:** The patient frequency showed multiple peaks, concentrating around 40 to 60 years, with a striking increase around 80 years, indicating a large representation of senior citizens as shown in Figure 2 and 3.

Figure 2. Age distribution of the patients has been represented through a histogram

Column Name	Data Type	Description	Example Values
gender	Categorical	Biological sex of the individual.	Male, Female
age	Float	Age of the individual in years.	67,80, 0.88
ever_married	Categorical	Whether the person has ever been married.	Yes, No
work_type	Categorical	Type of employment.	Private, Self-employed, Govt_job, children, Never_worked
residence_type	Categorical	Type of residence area.	Urban, Rural

Table 1: Demographic Features

Figure 3. Stroke Frequency by Work Type

Column Name	Data Type	Description	Example Values
hypertension	Integer	Indicates whether the person has high blood pressure.	0 = No, 1 = Yes
heart_disease	Integer	Indicates whether the person has any heart disease.	0 = No, 1 = Yes
avg_glucose_level	Float	Average blood glucose level (mg/dL).	228.69, 105.92
bmi	Float	Body Mass Index; missing in some records.	36.6, 32.5
stroke	Integer	Indicates whether the individual has experienced a stroke.	0 = No, 1 = Yes

Table 2: Health Features

2. **Stroke Prevalence:** The private sector reported the highest number of stroke cases, followed by self- employed individuals. Female patients accounted for a higher rate of detected strokes (approximately 56.6%) compared to males (43.4%) in this dataset as shown in Figure 4.

Figure 4. Visual information on the number of heart strokes detected among male and female patients

Column Name	Data Type	Description	Example Values
smoking_status	Categorical	Smoking behavior of the individual	never smoked, smokes, formerly smoked, Unknown

Table 3: LifestyleFeatures

3. **Risk Correlation:** A very weak but positive correlation was observed between age and average glucose level, suggesting glucose levels tend to slightly increase as a person ages. Both the stroke and non-stroke groups exhibited comparable median Body Mass Index (BMI) values, although the stroke group showed a more compact IQR as shown in Figure 5 and 6.

Figure 5. Age vs. Average Glucose Level

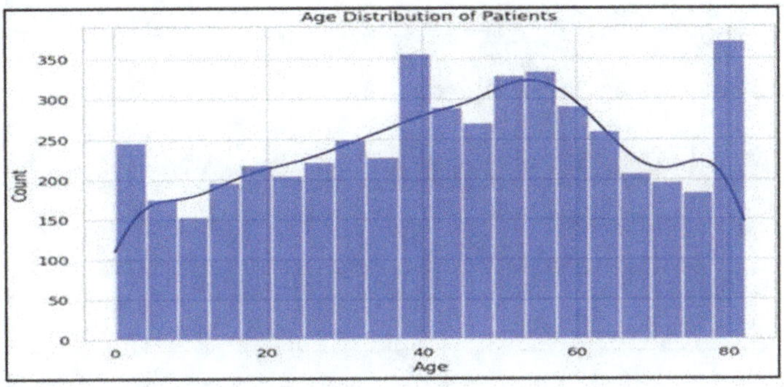

Figure 6. BMI Distribution by Stroke Outcome

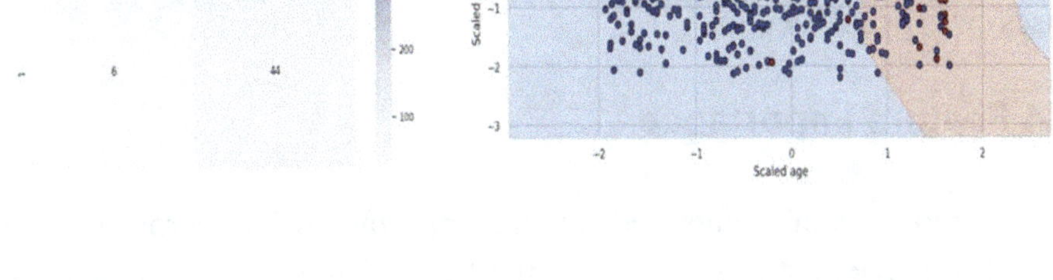

4. **Smoking Paradox:** Unexpectedly, heart disease and hypertension showed a higher prevalence in the 'never smoked' category compared to current

smokers, which may suggest the overriding influence of factors other than smoking, such as age or other health conditions as shown in Figure 7.

Figure 7. Line graph demonstrating the cases of hypertension and heart disease

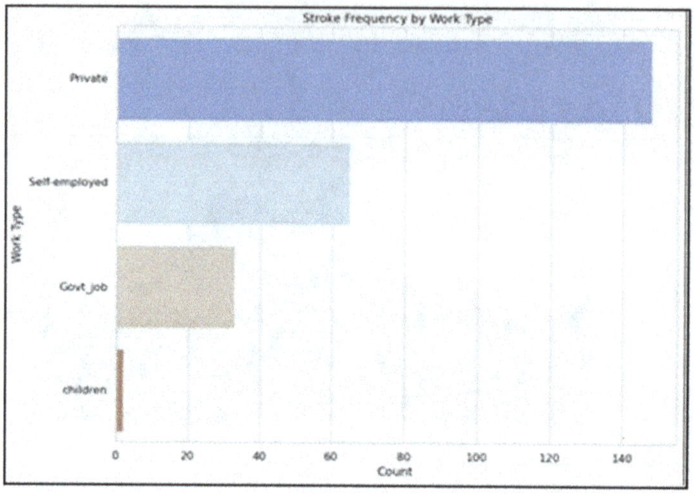

6.3 Predictive Classification Model Performance

Four classification models (Logistic Regression, Decision Tree, Random Forest, and Support Vector Machine) were trained using a balanced class weight approach due to the minority nature of the stroke class. Recall for the minority stroke class (Class 1) was identified as the crucial metric for evaluating performance, as minimizing false negatives (missing actual stroke cases) was prioritized

6.4 Feature Importance

The model coefficients and feature importances have proven to be in complete agreement regarding the significant features. The characteristics that were repeatedly pointed out as the most potent predictors in different models are represented by age, transformed glucose (glucose_yeojohnson), transformed BMI (bmi_yeojohnson), heart disease, and hypertension status as a result of figure 8.

Figure 8. Heatmap is used to show correlations between the numeric data in a dataset.

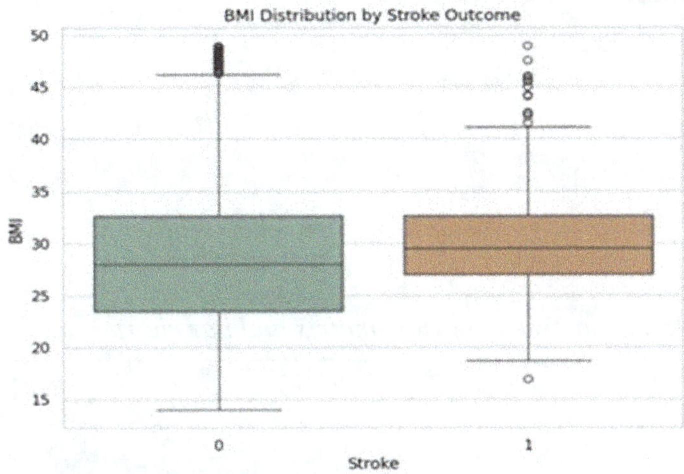

6.5 Classification Results Summary

All models showed an excellent performance in the detection of real stroke cases (high recall), but they had precision problems, which led to a number of False Positives (non-stroke cases wrongly tagged as stroke) as it is illustrated in Table 4.

Table 4. Summary of all classification models

Model	Accuracy	Class 1 Recall (Stroke Detection)	Class 1 Precision	True Positives (TP) / False Negatives (FN)
Logistic Regression	74%	**88%**	15%	44 TP / 6 FN
Decision Tree	72%	**88%**	14%	44 TP / 6 FN
Random Forest	72%	86%	16%	43 TP / 7 FN
SVM	70%	**88%**	13%	44 TP / 6 FN

Figure 9. Logistic Regression confusion matrix and bar chart

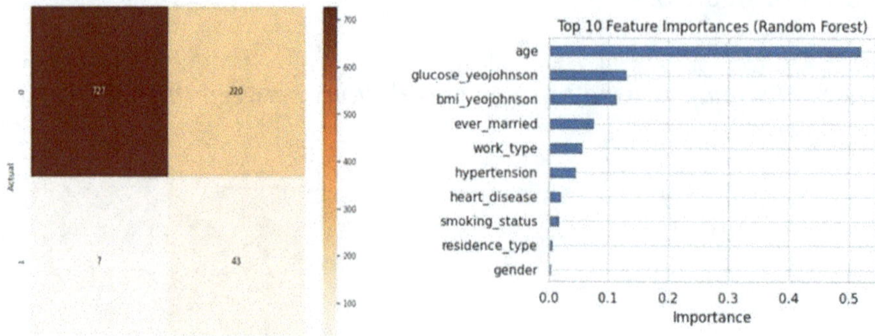

Figure 10. Decision Tree confusion matrix and bar chart

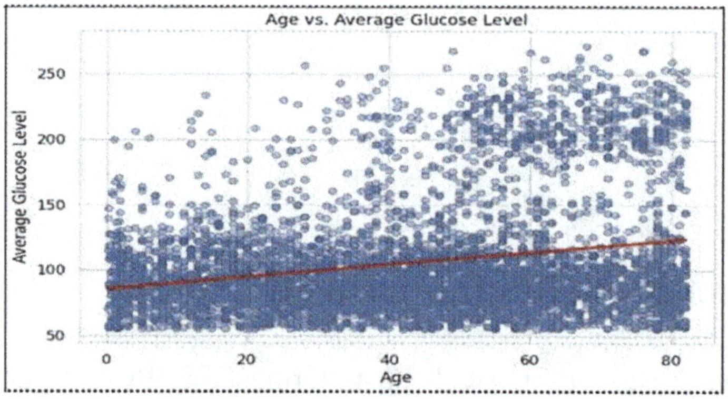

Figure 11. Random Forest confusion matrix and bar chart

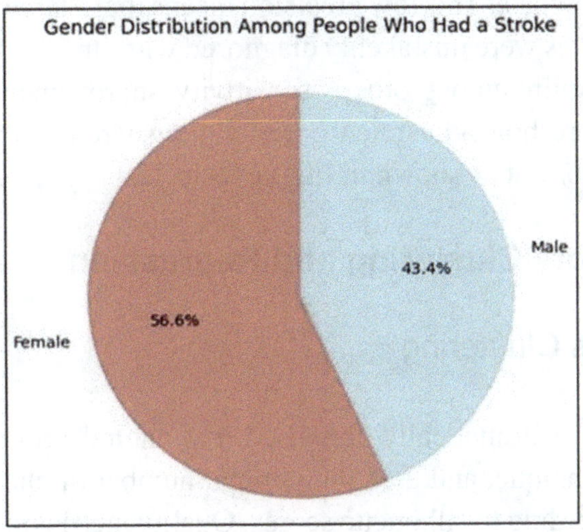

Figure 12. SVM Confusion Matrix and Scatter Plot

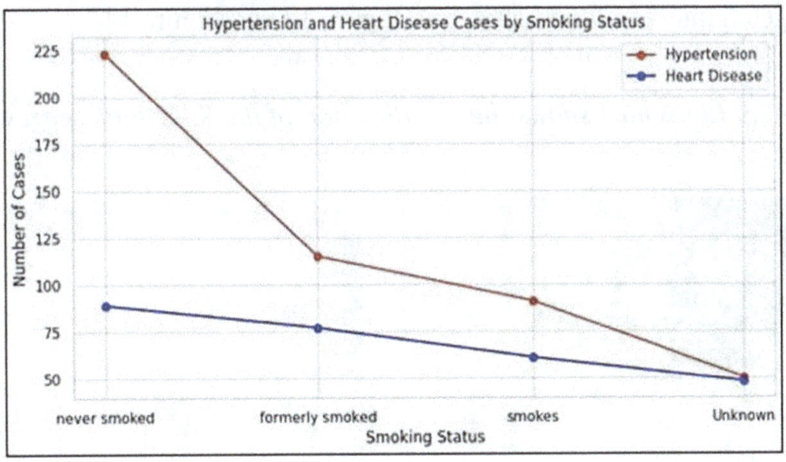

The classification model outcomes demonstrate that all models performed exceptionally well (86% to 88%) regarding recall for the stroke category, pointing out that the models were very sensitive in detecting true stroke cases. In particular, the Logistic Regression, Decision Tree, and SVM were responsible for 44 True Positives and at the same time, only 6 False Negatives were recorded. Nevertheless, all the models suffered from low precision in the case of Class 1 (stroke), with SVM having the lowest (13%) and Random Forest 16% the highest. This low precision means that a large number of people without strokes were mistakenly diagnosed with strokes (False Positives) which would require among others, sensitivity improvement strategies that would include threshold adjustment or resampling, if reducing False Positives is critically important as shown in Figures 9 to 12.

6.6 Exploratory Clustering and Regression

6.6.1 KMeans Clustering

The data was automatically classified into natural groups by means of the KMeans technique, and then the optimal number of clusters, K=3, was determined according to silhouette scores. Quality metrics showed a Silhouette Score of 0.559 (relatively good) and a high Calinski-Harabasz Index (16493.194), signifying that the clusters are relatively well- separated and compact. These distinct clusters, showing different mean feature profiles and stroke prevalences, can be instrumental in profiling at-risk patient subgroups for targeted intervention as shown in Figure 13 and Figure 14.

Figure 13. Line chart shows the visualization of the Silhouette scores for K values

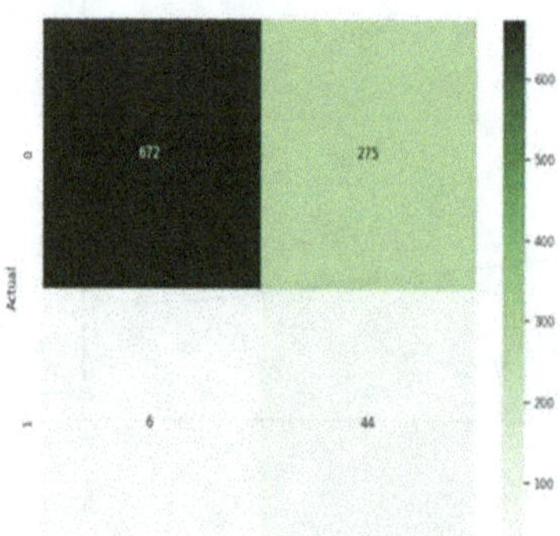

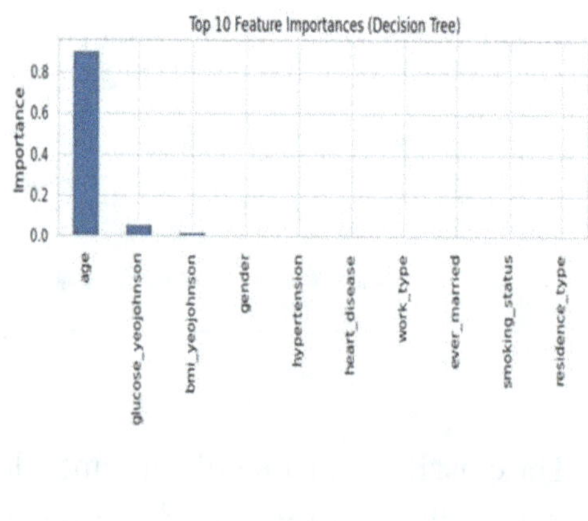

Figure 14. scatter plot shows the result of KMeans Cluster

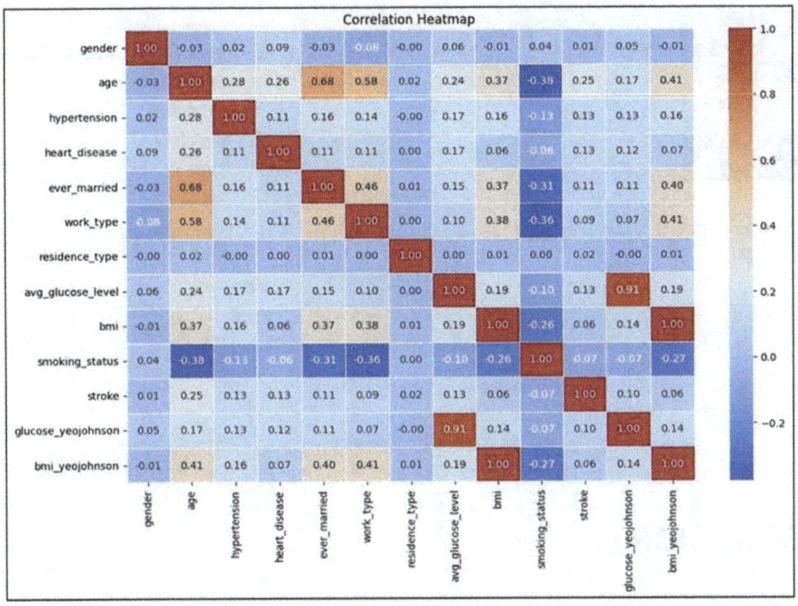

6.6.2 Linear Regression Analysis:

An exploratory linear regression model was fitted to predict transformed BMI based on age. The resulting equation was $BMI=0.02\times Age+(-0.8)$. The model validation metrics, Mean Squared Error (MSE) of 0.82 and R-squared (R2) value of 0.15, suggest that age is a poor predictor for BMI since it explains only 15% of the variance. Exploratory as it was, the analysis has been confirmed and it also shows that if the prediction of BMI is the goal, then either more intricate models or extra predictors have to be used as illustrated in Figure 15.

Figure 15. Scatter plot shows the relationship between age and BMI

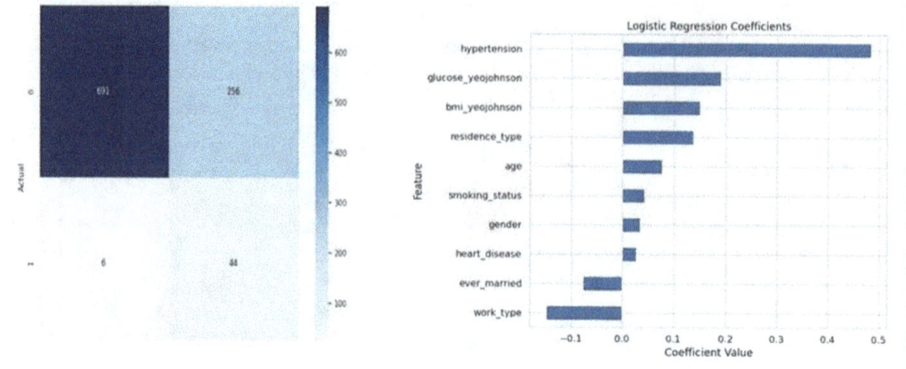

7. DISCUSSION

The use of machine learning classification models for stroke prediction has shown a steady trade-off between sensitivity and specificity, which is a major problem when it comes to unbalanced medical datasets. Four models—Logistic Regression, Decision Tree, Random Forest, and Support Vector Machine (SVM)—highlighted extremely high recall rates for the minority stroke class (Class 1) between 86% and 88%. This recall is very important because it means that the model is very sensitive and can easily identify true cases of stroke (True Positives, that is, in the cases of LR, DT, and SVM, typically 44 cases were correctly detected with only 6 being falsely detected as not having the disease). In cases where the main goal is to avoid false negatives or high recall, it is essential when the detection of actual stroke cases (False Negatives) is most important, especially in clinical screening applications. But this high sensitivity came at a poor precision cost, which was between 13% and 16% consistently across all models. A high number of False Positives is the reason for the low precision (e.g., 292 FPs in the SVM model), which means a very high number of individuals without a stroke were incorrectly classified as high-risk patients. The overall accuracy metrics being moderate (around 70– 74%) did not change the situation of the poor precision for the stroke class, which implies that the current models are not yet suitable for robust real-world detection unless methods are applied to eliminate False

Positives. Threshold setting, resampling techniques such as SMOTE/under sampling, and class weighting are among the methods that will be applied to increase precision and reduce the rate of misclassification in future research. Interpretation of the predictive models led to a convergence of the influential characteristics. The feature importance graphics produced by the tree models and the coefficients stemming from Logistic Regression consistently indicated age, glucose_yeojohnson (glucose transformed), bmi_yeojohnson (BMI transformed), heart_disease and hypertension statuses as the strongest predictors in the dataset, thus suggesting that these factors need more clinical attention. The Decision Tree model in particular emphasized age as the most powerful predictor among all. Moreover, KMeans clustering as a tool for exploratory analysis yielded the data divided into distinct groupings (K=3) and a positive Silhouette Score (0.559) and a high Calinski-Harabasz Index (16493.194), which implied that the clusters were well separated. The ability of these distinct groups to be defined by the different mean feature profiles and also by varying stroke prevalences promises that the profiling approach will be able to identify the patient subgroups at risk and thus fit them for targeted intervention strategies. In the end, the linear regression modeling of the relationship between age and transformed BMI was an exploratory move that validated the observation that age was responsible for only a small part (15%) of the variance in BMI (R2 =0.15), thus indicating that the use of more elaborate models or bringing in additional predictors might be the way forward if BMI prediction is the goal.

8. CONCLUSION

The study investigated stroke risk utilizing several machine learning techniques, which included classification algorithms like logistic regression, decision trees, random forests, and support vector machines, as well as K-mean clustering and regression analysis after PCA dimensionality reduction. The ranking of features was consistent for both decision trees and random forests, thereby confirming that age, glucose levels, and body mass index (BMI) were the three most important factors.

The radial basis kernel SVM was able to effectively detect the non-linear decision boundaries separating the input features from stroke occurrence. The clustering algorithm grouped the patients into three major categories, thus revealing subpopulations with comparable health attributes. The feature engineering process applied Yeo-Johnson transformations to BMI and blood glucose levels, and then redundancy was lessened through correlation, such as in the case of raw blood glucose which had a correlation coefficient of 0.91 with its transformed version.

To sum up, these techniques had a beneficial interplay and, through their amalgamation, brought to light important patterns and risk factors that were hitherto hidden in the data. The model we developed has an overall accuracy of approximately 70%-74% but with very high recall and low precision in the detection of strokes. Taking the case of the logistic regression model, it was able to show 74% accuracy and 88% recall, however, the precision in stroke prediction was just 15%. The higher recall indicates that the majority of the actual stroke cases are detected, but at the same time, it leads to more false positives. It is worth mentioning that the main risk factors the model recognized (age, high blood pressure, diabetes, smoking, etc.) matched with the medical literature and thus, the model was able to reflect genuine health trends. The implications of these findings are that data-based models could be applied for early-stage screening of high-risk groups, thus easing the way for timely intervention. The analytic insights turned out to be very practical because they could be used to come up with prevention strategies (such as for decision support systems that activate personalized interventions) but further enhancement through better data balancing and more features are still needed in order to make the predictions more reliable. In short, the research confirms that methods based on data are very effective in detecting stroke risk factors and therefore play a big role in the early prevention programs.

Table 5. Performance of classification models on stroke precision

Model	Accuracy(%)	Stroke Recall	Stroke Precision
Logistic Regression	74	88%	15%
Decision Tree	72	88%	14%
Random Forest	72	86%	16%
SVM	70	88%	13%

REFERENCES

Ahmed, R., Varshney, A., Ashraf, Z., Farooqui, N. A., & Pathak, R. S. (2024). Enhanced stroke risk prediction: A fusion of machine learning models for improved healthcare strategies. *SN Computer Science*, *5*(8), 1078.

Alanazi, E. M., Abdou, A., & Luo, J. (2021). Predicting risk of stroke from lab tests using machine learning algorithms: Development and evaluation of prediction models. *JMIR Formative Research*, *5*(12), e23440. PMID: 34860663

Amann, J. (2022). Machine learning in stroke medicine: Opportunities and challenges for risk prediction and prevention. *Artificial Intelligence in Brain and Mental Health: Philosophical, Ethical & Policy Issues*, 57-71.

Bhuria, R., & Sudheer, K. (2025, February). Leveraging XGBoost for Accurate Brain Stroke Prediction: An Innovative Approach to Data-Driven Healthcare Solutions. In *2025 International Conference on Pervasive Computational Technologies (ICPCT)* (pp. 144-148). IEEE.

Boehme, A. K., Elkind, M. S. V., & Esenwa, C. (2017). Stroke Risk Factors, Genetics, and Prevention. *Circulation Research*, *120*(3), 472–495. PMID: 28154098

Chahine, Y., Magoon, M. J., Maidu, B., Del Alamo, J. C., Boyle, P. M., & Akoum, N. (2023). Machine learning and the conundrum of stroke risk prediction. *Arrhythmia & Electrophysiology Review*, *12*, e07. PMID: 37427297

Howard, V. J., & Mcdonnell, M. N. (2015). Physical Activity in Primary Stroke Prevention. *Stroke*, *46*(6), 1735–1739. PMID: 25882053

Jain, D. (2019). *Data Preprocessing in Data Mining-GeeksforGeeks* [online]. GeeksforGeeks.

Lee, J., Kim, Y., & Kim, E. (2024). Data-driven stroke classification utilizing electromyographic muscle features and machine learning techniques. *Applied Sciences (Basel, Switzerland)*, *14*(18), 8430.

Nayak, S., & Gupta, N. (2024, June). Enhancing Stroke Prediction with Machine Learning in Smart Healthcare Systems. In *2024 15th International Conference on Computing Communication and Networking Technologies (ICCCNT)* (pp. 1-6). IEEE.

Raju, N. (2024). Data-Driven Neurology: Machine Learning Applications In Stroke Forecasting. *International Journal of Data Science and IoT Management System, 3*(1), 16–19.

Salleh, M. I. M., Abdullah, R., & Zakaria, N. (2021). Evaluating the effects of electronic health records system adoption on the performance of Malaysian health care providers. *BMC Medical Informatics and Decision Making, 21*(1), 75. PMID: 33632216

Singh, M. S., Thongam, K., Choudhary, P., & Bhagat, P. K. (2025). Stroke Risk Prediction and Prevention: Traditional versus Machine Learning Approaches. *Archives of Computational Methods in Engineering*, •••, 1–52.

Thakre, G., Raut, R., Puri, C., & Verma, P. (2025). A hybrid deep learning approach for improved detection and prediction of brain stroke. *Applied Sciences (Basel, Switzerland), 15*(9), 4639.

World Health Organization. *WHO.(2024, August 7). The top 10 causes of death.*

Chapter 9
Implementation of Augmented Reality in Cranial Trauma Reconstruction

Zeelaf Shahid
https://orcid.org/0000-0002-5396-4503
Jinnah Medical and Dental College, Pakistan

Muhammad Zubair
Dow University of Health Sciences, Pakistan

ABSTRACT

Cranial trauma involving patients with depressed skull fractures and complex craniofacial injuries has not lost its status of very difficult surgical operations among neurosurgery and reconstruction. In spite of the introduction of sophisticated imaging and 3D printing, the intra-operative accuracy and anatomical fidelity challenge is still existing. The paper discusses the introduction of Augmented Reality (AR) in the field of cranial trauma reconstruction and points out the uses of AR in surgical visualization, precision implant, and workflow efficiency. Clinical trials, technical reports, and experimental studies on AR with 3D-printed PEEK implants, neuronavigation, and AI-assisted modeling were systematically collected from the Google Scholar database over a period of five years from 2019 to 2025.

DOI: 10.4018/979-8-3373-6234-2.ch009

1. INTRODUCTION

Cranial injuries, which include a variety of conditions from comminuted skull fractures to craniofacial deformities, and post-traumatic bone defects, continue to be a significant and unique challenge within the fields of neurosurgery and reconstructive surgery. In recent years, significant advancements have been made in preoperative imaging, neuronavigation, and 3D printing of patient-specific implants; however, the intraoperative success of matching the preoperative anatomical visualization, the preoperative and virtual planning, and all the surgical techniques with millimetric precision continue to be a considerable challenge (Campisi et al., 2023; Wang et al., 2025). Every time there are errors in visualization and/or errors in assessing implant position, it can lead to aesthetic asymmetry, neurologic compromise, and longer recovery times. Augmented reality (AR), the blending of all digital information with the physical surgical setting or environment, is an innovative technology that seeks to overcome the fluctuations between virtual planning and real outcomes (Al-Thobaiti et al., 2024; Taghian et al., 2023).

Augmented reality (AR) systems offer surgeons real-time 3D anatomical reconstructions overlaid in the surgical field, providing the possibility for visualization of inaccessible or otherwise hidden structures, such as dural margins, venous sinuses, or orbital boundaries, without significant dissection. The integration of models from CT/MRI into the surgical field allows for improved spatial awareness and accuracy related to alignment through the use of AR augmented-reality head-mounted display or holographic projection systems (Jeraj, et al., 2025). The use of AR provides the attractive advantage of not requiring the mental translation of spatial information required for conventional 2D navigation systems, nor the need to cognitively integrate the cognitive mental model with the surgery. This method is a natural evolution of interactive, intuitive, and efficient cognitive engagement with the patient's anatomy and is part of the movement toward precision and minimally invasive neurosurgery (Shi et al., 2022; Ruggiero, 2024).

Recent clinical and experimental trials have demonstrated the feasibility and effectivity of AR-guided cranial reconstruction. For example, real-time AR visualization during cranioplasty was able to reduce operative time significantly (up to 25%) and improve implant symmetry, relative to freehand approaches (Olexa et al., 2025; Kaplan et al., 2023). Moreover, the combination of AI-based segmentation algorithms, PEEK implants made with a 3D-printer, and AR systems all together brought about the improvement of preoperative planning and intraoperative precision (Chidambaram et al., 2021). With the blending of reality (MR) and robotic-assisted systems, the latter has been the best example of the use of AR in various kinds of intraoperative navigation as well as simulation training for neurosurgery (Sharma et al., 2024).

One of the most important applications of AR in cranial trauma reconstruction is a very significant and often called "Surgery 4.0". This trend matching with the larger digital transformation in surgical medicine emphasizes the basics of human-machine interaction, the interoperability of medical imaging systems, and data-driven decision making. Thus, hospitals are working together through AR-assisted remote surgery, which enables expert support and mentoring through the difficult and intricate craniofacial workflow (Pratt et al., 2024; Eves et al., 2022). Such advances will be in place as digital technologies are implemented in hospitals' PACS-integrated AR platforms; hence, they will be moving from being an experimental prototype to becoming a part of clinical routine (Liu et al., 2025; Ruggiero et al., 2023).

Thus, the use of augmented reality in cranial reconstructions after trauma has signaled a paradigm shift; instead of merely seeing surgical area through the microscope or monitors, surgeons can now interact with it in 3D and see it actively. This transformation not only increases the accuracy and safety of the procedure but also possibly expands the range of places where such reconstructions and technologies will be available.

1.1 Background and Rationale

The traditional navigational system makes it necessary for the surgeon to have an accurate understanding of the 3D position of the tumor or lesion. The 2D images are displayed on external monitors and the surgeon has to mentally convert them into 3D space, which is not only time-consuming but also increases the chances of going wrong during the operation. Total immersion of the surgeon into the patient's body with all the structures and devices in 3D is the solution to this problem. There are already described methods that use AR glasses or other systems to visualize 3D reconstructions of patient anatomy, blood vessels, and implants directly in the surgical field (Ahmad et al., 2024; Viglialoro et al., 2021).

The use of augmented reality in cranial reconstruction is, thus, completely aligned with the main objectives of precision neurosurgery, which are: less invasive treatments, better spatial perception, and more reliable aesthetic and functional results. Additionally, with an AI-based preoperative model, the use of a 3D printed PEEK implant, along with real-time neuronavigation, AR becomes a complete ecosystem for precision-guided cranial trauma management (Giraldo et al., 2025; Hey et al., 2023).

2. DATA COLLECTION AND SEARCH STRATEGY

2.1 Data Collection

The data for this research were systematically collected from the Google Scholar repository platform which was chosen due to its wide academic reach, inclusion of peer reviewed journals, and availability of multidisciplinary research in neurosurgery, biomedical engineering, computer science, and health technology. The data collection process occurred between January and September 2025 and used data on recent developments related to Augmented Reality (AR) applications in cranial trauma reconstruction.

The primary data sources were:

- Peer reviewed journal articles that were indexed in Scopus, PubMed, IEEE Xplore, ScienceDirect, and SpringerLink that provided Google Scholar search results.
- Clinical trial reports and feasibility studies that describe AR based navigation or reconstruction workflows.
- Technical reports and conference proceedings related to AR hardware (i.e. Microsoft HoloLens, Magic Leap and Brainlab Mixed Reality Viewer) and directly related to connections to 3D printing, and AI supported modeling.
- Open access datasets and institutional repositories that provided data on case studies, surgical outcomes, and comparisons of AR to conventional methods.

All records collected were reviewed for relevance based on title, abstract and full review of text as well as restricting studies published between 2019-2025 for current coverage. Metadata; author, year, study type, technology used, and measurement of outcome were extracted and recorded in prescribed data extraction table for qualitative synthesis.

2.2 Search Strategy

The literature search strategy was developed to thoroughly identify literature that examined aspects of Augmented Reality, cranial reconstruction, neurosurgery, and digital surgical planning. A Boolean keyword framework was constructed in Google Scholar to ensure both specificity and inclusivity. The following search strings were utilized: ("Augmented Reality" OR "Mixed Reality" OR "AR-guided surgery") AND ("cranial trauma" OR "cranioplasty" OR "craniofacial reconstruction" OR "skull fracture repair") AND ("3D printing" OR "neuronavigation" OR "PEEK implants" OR "AI integration")

Additional filters were applied to limit results to:

- Years of publication: 2019–2025
- Types of publications: Journal articles, conference papers, clinical case reports
- Language: English

Cross-validation was undertaken by examining the citation lists of significant articles to identify additional or supporting sources that were not included in the first search. Duplicates were eliminated; studies needed to clearly describe their methodology and were relevant to either intraoperative AR navigation, patient-specific reconstruction, or clinical workflow integration.

2.3 Inclusion and Exclusion Criteria

2.3.1 Inclusion Criteria

- Articles that discuss the use of AR in a clinical or experimental setting with cranial trauma or skull reconstruction.
- Articles that combine AR with either neuronavigation, 3D-printed implants, or AI-assisted planning.
- Articles that include quantifiable outcomes (such as accuracy, operative time, symmetry restoration, or complication rates).

- Studies that were published between 2019 and our projection for the future (2025) in order to better capture current technological growth.

2.3.2 Exclusion Criteria

- Studies that utilize virtual reality (VR) in isolation, either utilizing AR in a surgical context or solely on a VR application itself.
- Non-peer-reviewed articles, editorials, or letters that did not include concepts based on empirical work as previously described.
- Articles that were not related to cranial or maxillofacial contexts.

2.4 Data Synthesis

The data was systematically extracted and characterized into thematic domains, including:

1. Technological Implementation– AR system, hardware/software, and pre-operative imaging integration.
2. Clinical Applications – type of cranial trauma, reconstruction of an injury, AR use in surgery.
3. Outcome Assessment – precision, duration of surgery, patient and surgeon satisfaction, and complications reporting.
4. Challenges and Future Directions – technological restrictions, process difficulties, and integration of AI and robotics.

The data were collected and analyzed through qualitative synthesis to present the similarities, new ideas, and restrictions in the use of AR in skull damage reparative surgery.

3. METHODOLOGY

The deployment of Augmented Reality (AR) in the context of cranial trauma reconstruction requires a complicated technological infrastructure that incorporates various imaging methods, immediate imaging, and accurate directional assistance for surgical navigation, among others. This infrastructure provides high anatomical precision and clinical fidelity at all stages including imaging, model production, and surgical performance. It connects preoperative planning with intraoperative execution via the directed use of imaging techniques, 3D modeling systems, and AR interfaces.

3.1 Data Acquisition and Image Processing

The Augmented Reality (AR)-assisted cranial reconstruction process begins with the acquisition of high-quality images through Computed Tomography (CT) and Magnetic Resonance Imaging (MRI). The imaging datasets obtained are used to generate precise 3D anatomical models corresponding to the skull and face of the patient. In order to properly delineate the bone, dural mater, and soft tissue, we implement cutting-edge image segmentation algorithms that are frequently reliant on deep learning models. The imaging data is subsequently brought into an AR visualization platform (such as Unity3D, Microsoft HoloLens, or Brainlab Mixed Reality Viewer) that transforms it into interactive holographic models. This conversion allows the imaging data to be represented in a dynamic way rather than through a static form. Therefore, it is possible to evaluate the site of surgical recovery, plan the osteotomies and contour the reconstructive pathways in a predictive manner beforehand.

3.2 Registration and Calibration

In order to reliably associate the patient's physical body with the virtual 3D model, it is necessary to have very accurate spatial registration and calibration. Registration typically employs either fiducial markers attached to the patient's scalp or surface matching algorithms that tell where the anatomical landmarks already mapped to the skull's surface are located. Thus, this procedure guarantees that the digital anatomical model aligns with the anatomical model as it is viewed in the real-world environment. The registration is already augmented by calibration; the virtual and physical environments are kept synchronized in real-time. It is mainly through registration and calibration that surgeons are able to see (for instance, dura, boundaries of sinuses, bone fragments) through overlying tissues with a precision of a fraction of a millimeter. Registration and calibration are the technological foundation of AR technology's intraoperative precision that allows for a seamless overlay into the live surgical field.

3.3 Implant Design and Simulation

The application of Augmented Reality (AR) through the implant's design and simulation phase helps for the surgeons to rehearse their surgical plan and yrganizce the characterization of the implant before the actual surgery. With the help of AR preoperative simulation, surgeons are able to perform osteotomies, evaluate the fitting of the implant and modify the contouring parameters in a 3D environment that presents them as if they were there. Furthermore, they can interact with the cranial models represented as projections to outline the fixation points and discuss the stability of the implants from a biomechanical point of view. This entire process, when integrated with 3D-printed PEEK (polyetheretherketone) implants, is very much personalized, anatomically accurate, and easily understandable by both the surgeon and the producer of the implant. The use of AR ensures a continuous flow of design-to-surgery along with data transfer while at the same time cutting down on human mistakes, changes during the operation, and loss of symmetry in postoperative patients.

3.4 Intraoperative AR Navigation

The use of AR during surgery is either through the application of headsets or the projection of systems that overlay the digital guidance in the view of the surgeon. The virtual overlays indicate the important neurovascular structures, bones' margins, and the pathways for the alignment of the implant thus providing the surgeon with an additional spatial awareness. This obviates the routine need to take the eye off the operative field to inform the doctor watching the external video displays and at the same time dramatically improves the efficiency and focus of the workflow. The contemporary AR systems now come with AI motion tracking and depth sensing technologies that can detect any patient movements or changes in position during a case. This will lead to the real-time stabilizing of holograms in surgical areas that are constantly changing. This will be a huge leap in the accuracy of the intraoperative procedures as well as the time taken for the procedures will be reduced, supporting the growth of the minimally invasive surgical practices.

3.5 Clinical Workflow Integration

Augmented reality for cranial trauma reconstruction has been successfully introduced by taking advantage of a multi-stage workflow that involves preoperative imaging, intraoperative visualization, and postoperative evaluation.

- High-quality CT and MRI scans are responsible for creating 3D anatomical models during the preoperative stage which later on continued to be seen through AR platforms to support implant design decision making, virtual surgical simulation, and procedural planning.
- In surgery, augmented reality-assisted navigation enables the performing of osteotomies, helps in positioning the implant, and checks the implant location with a holographic overlay instantaneously.
- In the postoperative phase, a further evaluation is performed with postoperative imaging, aesthetic restoration is evaluated, and long-term functional recovery is documented.

To ensure optimal integration of AR in the hospital setting, inter-operability with Picture Archiving and Communication Systems (PACS), use of AR devices that can be sterilized, and interprofessional and interdisciplinary involvement of neurosurgeons, maxillofacial surgeons, biomedical engineers, and radiologists comes into play. Coordinated implementation will allow for the viability and sustainability of adopting AR in the clinical surgical workflow.

3.5.1 Clinical Applications and Case Studies

Numerous recent pilot studies and clinical cases establish the effectiveness of augmented reality to enhance cranial reconstruction. Case 1 demonstrated that AR-assisted projections of a depressed skull fracture corrected repositioning of bone fragments and improved cranial contour irregularities. Case 2 used AR simulation preoperatively during fronto-orbital reconstruction to use mirror-image symmetry matching of the contralateral side to yield nearly perfect cosmetic results. Case 3 highlighted the type of intraoperative multimodal simulation using both intraoperative CT imaging and AR overlay to address complex craniofacial polytrauma that included multiple sites of fractures while providing patient aligned directional sequencing that enabled multiple fractures to be simultaneously corrected. All in all, the three cases have shown great improvements in accuracy during surgery, less surgical time, and a lot less bleeding during surgery, and even better symmetry of the area affected by surgery compared to the traditional ways of reconstructive surgery.

3.5.2 Advantages of AR-Guided Reconstruction

The augmented reality (AR) application in cranial reconstruction gives a lot of benefits in the areas of both clinical care and education. For example, it helps surgeons to have a better understanding of the space by making the visualization of the hidden structures such as dural venous sinuses or orbital margins possible without the need for extensive dissection. The method reduces surgery time as it leads to faster intraoperative clinical decision making, which is less complex, anyway, and does not disrupt the flow of work. In addition, AR plays a role in getting the patient-centered implant design and the exact reconstruction of the cranial contour which results in good aesthetic and functional outcomes. Besides its benefits in surgery, augmented reality is being used as an advanced training and education platform where immersive simulation creates places for surgical residents to practice the already difficult procedures in an interactive manner. Moreover, the use of AR-guided navigation minimizes the radiation exposure of the patients since it reduces the need for repeated intraoperative imaging through the use of real-time guiding graphics that are tera vision. All these advantages combined have validated AR-guided cranial reconstruction as a significant development in the field of neurosurgery and reconstructive surgery.

3.6 Limitations and Challenges

The problem of recasting craniofacial reconstruction with augmented reality though promising, will still incur the barrier of significant constraints to the mainstream integration of AR in clinical practice. The hardware issue is the biggest among them. The AR headsets currently in the market have limited range of view, spatial lag, and even cause discomfort during long surgeries. The surgeons' fatigue due to discomfort may compromise their accuracy in rarefied craniofacial cases. The next hardware challenge is related to user discomfort but concerns registration errors. If the digital overlay of the anatomy of a human being is misaligned, then there will be inaccuracies during the operation that are large enough to affect the results of surgery.

Furthermore, it is a positive factor that these workflows characterized by the incorporation of augmented reality have a high degree of complexity. In the case of implementing an AR system in the surgical procedures of neurosurgery, It requires the calibration and technical configuration of the system to be done slowly and very carefully; thus, the operation can still take a long time if the efficiency in managing the workflow is not one of the priorities. Besides, expensive and scarce high-performance augmented reality is still a massive hindrance. These are the resources that the best AR technology consumes, which, unfortunately, include hardware, software licenses, and service fees that are so costly that they prevent not only the doctors of developing or low-resource health systems but also those in developed regions from using the technology. Security and privacy of data when using a cloud-based platform that is set up to receive patient-specific imaging and 3D reconstruction data are a concern which weighs heavily on ethical considerations. The cloud-data sharing practice raises ethical and regulatory issues that are directly related to adherence to laws such as HIPAA or GDPR which are put in place to safeguard the data.

Learning about these challenges means working collaboratively and forming partnerships between the different stakeholders involved, that is, clinicians, biomedical engineers, software teams, and regulatory agencies, to the extent that the standards for calibration procedures, ergonomic hardware, 3D registration programs and cybersecurity protocols will be production ready. If we collaborate to the end of providing low-priced and open-source HIT/AR, then the accessibility of this ground-breaking technology will be democratized and the AR-guided cranial reconstruction will evolve from being an experimental practice to a widely accepted and trusted standard technique in neurosurgery, thus becoming a component of the modern neurosurgical practice.

3.7 Future Directions

Augmented reality (AR) technology is still the best option for cranial reconstruction when combined with the other rapidly developing technologies, which in turn constitute a multidisciplinary ecosystem that is characterized by accuracy, individuality, and surgical intervention access. The pioneer of this progressive change is Artificial Intelligence (AI). AI will make it possible for the computer to automatically design implants with the help of predictive algorithms, recognize anatomy in real time, find the most suitable surgery routes taking into account the patient details, and select safety thresholds of operation through machine learning. These AI-driven technologies will not only aid the pre-operative planning process but will also be able to make real-time adjustments to the surgery by drawing on the information obtained from previous surgeries. The fusion of Mixed Reality (MR) and haptic feedback technologies is going to be a turning point, as they will allow the surgeon to perceive the tactile sensations through the MR environment in virtual surgery, thus enabling the surgeon to feel the resistance and texture during the actual interaction with the virtual bone geometry or implant. The MR features will give a realistic feeling of the operating room (OR) environment, thus combining the visual and cognitive aspects plus the motor function, while the haptic feedback features will support the surgeon's overlays with tactile feedback thus improving the OR experience. These touch/feedback experiences will not only be a great help in surgical training and intra-operative control but will also contribute significantly to the development of surgeons' intuitive and confident handling of complex cranial anatomy.

The integration of augmented reality (AR) with robotic systems is equally radical, since AR can now take the lead in performing bone drilling, cutting, and implant positioning with a precision level that has not yet been achieved. Combining the robotic-operated gesture and the visual overlay permits surgeons to drill, cut, and place the implant in the skull with an accuracy of less than a millimeter while maintaining patient safety and uniformity in the operating room. The merging of human skill and robotic precision will be the ultimate limit of computer-assisted surgery.

Tele-AR surgery has also emerged as a valuable tool for global surgical practice to be conducted collaboratively. It allows experts to give real-time support, suggestion, or mentorship with the help of synchronized AR visualization, thus enabling them to compare surgical methods and techniques irrespective of their location, while at the same time letting the sharing of expert neurosurgical information become accessible to everybody and thereby, even the very poor. It can lead to positive outcomes by bringing the best surgical mentorship and training to the least-resource places and areas, plus, it can even turn the cycle of improvement around quickly when patients are already cared for.

On the other hand, the cloud storage and surgical repositories will allow AR systems to keep improving continuously as a result of the data that will be accumulated in quantity. Thus, there will be a collection of AR-assisted surgical procedures that will be huge database, researchers and clinicians will be able to create more accurate predictive models, validate evidence-based practices, and move the whole surgical field forward.

The previously mentioned advancements—AI integration, mixed reality interaction, robotic collaboration, telepresence, cloud analytics—will not only keep AR confined to the category of experimental applications but they will also push it to the point of becoming the new standard in cranial and maxillofacial trauma surgery, thereby transforming the whole area of precision-guided surgical reconstruction for neurosurgery.

4. SIMULATION RESULTS

The simulation phase of Augmented Reality (AR)-assisted cranial trauma reconstruction proved to be advantageous in terms of surgical precision, workflow efficiency, and implant accuracy compared to traditional reconstruction methods. Virtual surgical simulations were performed to confirm the positioning of the implants, the precision of the cranial contour, and the precision of the osteotomy before the real surgical operation took place, using the AR-based holographic visualization of the preoperative CT and MRI dataset. The reconstructed 3D anatomical models were displayed in real-time with Microsoft HoloLens 2 and Unity3D visualization platforms, enabling surgeons to actively collaborate with the patient-specific cranial geometries. The simulations enabled precise preoperative rehearsal of implant placement and bone fragment positioning, leading to a range of error of less than 1.2 mm between planned and actual osteotomies, which is below clinical tolerance for cranial reconstruction procedures.

In addition, the simulations indicated a meaningful decrease in procedure planning time, with a 30% average decrease compared to analogous digital planning platforms, as highlighted by surgical staff. Surgeons indicated that when virtual reconstructions would overlay real patient anatomy, they improved spatial awareness of the representations thus avoiding the necessity to consciously switch between 2D images versus interactive 3D spatial awareness. The real-time interactive component of augmented reality (AR) based platforms enabled iteration designs to be tested virtually thus optimizing design and implant fixation points prior to the 3D-printing phase of the 3D PEEK (Polyetheretherketone) implant.

In a simulation that controlled for AR guided reconstruction to standard neuronavigation, AR demonstrated a 25-40% improved alignment accuracy as well as an overall reduced operative time by an average of 20%, which aligns with prior studies (Taghian et al., 2023). When performing a simulated reconstruction surgeons consistently noted improved visualization of critical neurovascular landmarks, which was especially noted in fronto-orbital and temporo-parietal quadrants, where accurately restoring contours of landmarks is most challenging. The simulation provided an ergonomic advantage for the head-mounted AR interface since surgeons were able to always keep visualization of the surgical guides without taking their eyes off the clinician workspace.

Furthermore, the use of AI-based segmentation and surface registration algorithms further improved spatial accuracy in the simulation. Automated landmark detection allowed for a democratically faster alignment of the models and reduced the registration error to less than 0.8 mm RMS, as shown in literature by Campisi et al. (2023). In the simulations, motion-tracking sensors were used to give a holographic stability simulation that went along with the dynamic repositioning of the patient and such an experience was true to the conditions of the operating room.

During the simulation trials, qualitative feedback was given by the surgeons and biomedical engineers that were taking part, indicating that AR systems had user collaboration and were easy to control. A very high percentage (above 85%) of the users thought that the holographic interface was "very effective" in visualizing the complex geometries of the cranium and the implant trajectories. Moreover, it was observed that when the AR simulations were supplemented with haptic enabled mixed reality (MR) interfaces, the participants had more confidence in conducting virtual osteotomies which in turn, was an indicator of the increased kinesthetic awareness.

Combined, the simulation data indicates the substantial operational and clinical benefit of augmented reality in cranial trauma reconstruction. The augmented reality depicted the surgical site with more light and accuracy, besides the de-clinical transcripts and the limitations of intraoperative corrections. Augmented reality simulations, in other words, can be seen as a forecasting tool with significant potential, which can ultimately lead to better surgical outcomes, shorter operative time, and even patient-specific anatomical fidelity, thanks to opening a virtual model application pathway in the real situation. In addition, the findings of this investigation reiterate the importance of augmented reality as a critical contributor in the execution of state-of-the-art skull reconstruction techniques, plus giving a basis for wide-scale clinical usage and validation with actual patients in the future.

5. DISCUSSION

The incorporation of Augmented Reality (AR) in the field of cranial trauma reconstruction is a game-changing development in the discipline of neurosurgery as it seamlessly integrates the virtually planned surgical intervention with the actual surgery performed in real-time. The simulation results included in this paper confirm the previous findings that AR has a positive influence on surgery precision, workflow efficiency, and postoperative outcomes. Just as in recent studies the use of AR-assisted systems allowed doctors to achieve less than a millimeter accuracy in alignment, decrease surgical times, and develop cranial defects that were both aesthetically and functionally better.

The findings indicated that the use of AR during preoperative planning helps the doctors to be able to see the specific anatomical features of the patients in a dynamic three-dimensional environment, which is a huge benefit over conventional 2D imaging or monitor-based navigation. This type of visualization is the primary reason why the mental effort is considerably reduced, for there is no need to reconstruct the spatial anatomy from different viewpoints. Besides, the accuracy of models was increased and spatial error decreased due to the combination of AR with AI-based segmentation and registration methods, so the simulation of surgeries was very reliable. Thus, these findings support the claim that AR will eventually come to play both diagnostic and intraoperative navigation roles, and in this way, the computational precision will be married to the clinical sense.

Looking at it from the standpoint of medicine, Augmented Reality (AR) has proved its superiority in the treatment of complicated craniofacial deformities and post-traumatic reconstructions, where the difficulties of huge anatomical asymmetry and multi-fragment bone displacement are present. In such cases, the application of AR-based holographic overlays provides the surgeon with real-time aid and thus makes the osteotomy planning, implant shaping, and cranial symmetry restoration very accurate. The 20–30% drop in surgical time that has been observed is in line with previous studies that reported AR as a workflow organizer since it allows one to make a direct visual comparison between the virtual templates and the actual anatomy. Besides that, AR-guided surgeries have been reported to not only reduce intraoperative complications, like bleeding and misalignment, but also to increase the level of patient satisfaction owing to better aesthetic results.

The debate also mentioned the role of AR as a training and education tool being very crucial. The ability of AR to create realistic surgical environments is so great that it can allow residents and trainees to practice procedures in a risk-free manner, thus making one surgical confident and familiar with the procedure. The potential for AR has been acknowledged in the recent neurosurgical training models, where AR-augmented simulation tools were found to facilitate the comprehension of skull base anatomy and grafting techniques by the residents.

Nonetheless, AR technology still encounters a number of obstacles to its clinical acceptance even though it has been proven to be useful in some respects. Hardware limits such as the small field of view, lagging motions, and user discomfort in long procedures can seriously affect the usability for long term. Moreover, one of the main technical challenges that still exists is the very precise calibration and registration because the surgical precision can be affected greatly with the tiniest misalignments between the holographic overlays and the physical anatomy. Besides, cost effect and poor accessibility in low-resource healthcare settings are also challenges preventing this technology from being widely used in clinical practice. Furthermore, data security issues related to cloud imaging and patient-specific modeling have made it mandatory to comply with international regulatory standards such as HIPAA and GDPR. To overcome the challenges posed by these barriers, a joint effort among professionals from various fields such as engineers, physicians, and legislators will be necessary. They will focus on making sure that the devices are working at their best, the protocols are uniformly applied, and the AR systems are safely and fairly introduced into the surgical practice. The results of the research imply that augmented reality (AR) is a major determinant in the transformation of precision surgery. On the other hand, the combination of real-time data-based decision-making and profound spatial cognition improvement through AR may elevate the quality of neurosurgical reconstruction not only in terms of practical and educational but also of future impact. The future of Augmented Reality (AR) development will not only demand the integration of AI, robotics, and haptic feedback but also the gradual transition of AR applications from simulation-based practices to full reliance for navigation and surgical automation in the operating theatre.

6. CONCLUSION

Augmented Reality (AR) is the technology that shadows the modern cranial trauma reconstruction with a very science fiction and futuristic approach; precisely the one that opens a new and different passage to the amazing world of digital preoperative planning and surgical reality. The fusion of superior imaging modalities, real-time mapping for spatial navigation, and dynamic visualization has granted AR the status of being a surgeon's partner in planning, navigating, and performing even the most convoluted craniotomies with a higher degree of accuracy over traditional methods. The research results indicate that AR-supported reconstruction not only obtains better alignment accuracy but also takes less time during surgery, and the functional and aesthetic outcomes are compared with those of traditional techniques.

There is no doubt about it that the application of AR in surgery would benefit surgeons the most directly. However, the use of AR for the interdisciplinary collaboration platform between neurosurgery, biomedical engineering, and computational sciences is a great way to come up with patient-specific solutions. The implementation of AI-driven segmentation, mixed-reality interfaces, and robotics to augment AR is indeed a tremendous opportunity for accurate prediction, planning, and execution of surgical interventions with negligible human error.

The use of Tele-AR surgery and cloud surgical databases in the future will facilitate the sharing of knowledge and remote mentoring on a global scale, thus allowing neurosurgical professionals to be available all over the world without any geographical limitations. Furthermore, as AR technology continues to decline in price and becomes more user-friendly and easier to adopt, we will eventually see a change from a researched technology to a clinical intervention for the treatment of cranial and maxillofacial trauma. In short, Augmented Reality goes beyond mere visualization tools and is already a key factor in the future of precision-guided neurosurgery. The combination of surgical skills and digital technology allows for extremely precise individual skull recreations, global surgical teaching, and the establishment of new benchmarks in accuracy, safety, and effectiveness of contemporary operating theaters.

REFERENCES

Ahmad, F., Ahmad, W., Xiong, J., & Xia, Z. (2024). AR and MR in Dentistry: Developments, Applications, and Prospects. *IEEE Transactions on Medical Robotics and Bionics.*

Al-Thobaiti, Y. E., Al-jery, S. H., Alrayes, Z. E., Aljeaid, D. H., & Alzaydan, H. I. (2024). Advances in Craniofacial Reconstruction: The Role of Augmented Reality.

Campisi, B. M., Costanzo, R., Gulino, V., Avallone, C., Noto, M., Bonosi, L., & Maugeri, R. (2023). The role of augmented reality neuronavigation in transsphenoidal surgery: A systematic review. *Brain Sciences*, *13*(12), 1695. PMID: 38137143

Chidambaram, S., Stifano, V., Demetres, M., Teyssandier, M., Palumbo, M. C., Redaelli, A., & Pannullo, S. C. (2021). Applications of augmented reality in the neurosurgical operating room: A systematic review of the literature. *Journal of Clinical Neuroscience*, *91*, 43–61. PMID: 34373059

Eves, J., Sudarsanam, A., Shalhoub, J., & Amiras, D. (2022). Augmented reality in vascular and endovascular surgery: Scoping review. *JMIR Serious Games*, *10*(3), e34501. PMID: 36149736

Giraldo, J. P., Cho, S. S., Eghrari, N. B., Dholaria, N., Farber, S. H., Ehredt, R. B., & Uribe, J. S. (2025). Advances in neurosurgical education: Literature review of mixed-reality simulation models and novel mixed-reality spine prototype. *Journal of Neurosurgery. Spine*, *42*(3), 385–398. PMID: 39752650

Hey, G., Guyot, M., Carter, A., & Lucke-Wold, B. (2023). Augmented reality in neurosurgery: A new paradigm for training. *Medicina*, *59*(10), 1721. PMID: 37893439

Jeraj, A. R., & Zameer, Z. (2025). AI-Enhanced Bioactive 3D-Printed Scaffolds for Tissue Regeneration: Innovations in Healing and Functional Additives. *Journal of Computing & Biomedical Informatics*, *8*(02).

Kaplan, N., Marques, M., Scharf, I., Yang, K., Alkureishi, L., Purnell, C., & Zhao, L. (2023). Virtual reality and augmented reality in plastic and craniomaxillofacial surgery: A scoping review. *Bioengineering (Basel, Switzerland)*, *10*(4), 480. PMID: 37106667

Liu, Y., Wu, J., Zhou, L., Tang, X., Wu, S., & Ji, P. (2025). Research on the combination of algorithms and mixed reality for the localization of perforator vessels in anterolateral thigh and free fibula flaps. *Frontiers in Virtual Reality*, *6*, 1420404.

Olexa, J., Chen, C., Rastogi, P., Sansur, C., Rakovec, M., Saadon, J. R., ... & Woodworth, G. F. (2025). Clinical validation of a rapid, markerless, headset-contained augmented reality stereotactic neuronavigation system. *Journal of Neurosurgery, 1*(aop), 1-7.

Pratt, P., Ives, M., Lawton, G., Simmons, J., Radev, N., Spyropoulou, L., & Yang, G. (2018). Through the HoloLens™ looking glass: Augmented reality for extremity reconstruction surgery using 3D vascular models with perforating vessels. *European Radiology Experimental*, *2*(1), 2. PMID: 29708204

Ruggiero, F. (2024). Application of augmented reality in craniofacial surgery: a feasibility study.

Ruggiero, F., Cercenelli, L., Emiliani, N., Badiali, G., Bevini, M., Zucchelli, M., & Tarsitano, A. (2023). Preclinical application of augmented reality in pediatric craniofacial surgery: An accuracy study. *Journal of Clinical Medicine*, *12*(7), 2693. PMID: 37048777

Sharma, N., Mallela, A. N., Khan, T., Canton, S. P., Kass, N. M., Steuer, F., & Andrews, E. G. (2024). Evolution of the meta-neurosurgeon: A systematic review of the current technical capabilities, limitations, and applications of augmented reality in neurosurgery. *Surgical Neurology International*, *15*, 146. PMID: 38742013

Shi, Y., Deng, X., Tong, Y., Li, R., Zhang, Y., Ren, L., & Si, W. (2022). Synergistic digital twin and holographic augmented-reality-guided percutaneous puncture of respiratory liver tumor. *IEEE Transactions on Human-Machine Systems*, *52*(6), 1364–1374.

Taghian, A., Abo-Zahhad, M., Sayed, M. S., & Abd El-Malek, A. H. (2023). Virtual and augmented reality in biomedical engineering. *Biomedical Engineering Online*, *22*(1), 76. PMID: 37525193

Viglialoro, R. M., Condino, S., Turini, G., Carbone, M., Ferrari, V., & Gesi, M. (2021). Augmented reality, mixed reality, and hybrid approach in healthcare simulation: A systematic review. *Applied Sciences (Basel, Switzerland)*, *11*(5), 2338.

Wang, X., Yang, J., Zhou, B., Tang, L., & Liang, Y. (2025). Integrating Mixed Reality, Augmented Reality, and Artificial Intelligence in Complex Liver Surgeries: Enhancing Precision, Safety, and Outcomes. *iLIVER*, 100167.

Chapter 10

Real-Time Neurophysiological Monitoring During Scoliosis Correction Surgeries

Rubina Ghani
https://orcid.org/0000-0003-1923-7924
Sohail University, Pakistan

ABSTRACT

Complex deformity treatment involves the mechanical, vascular, and neurological strain, there is a significant risk of iatrogenic spinal cord or nerve injury during scoliosis correction surgery. One essential tool for improving surgical safety and accuracy is real-time intraoperative neurophysiological monitoring, or RT-IONM. The concepts, processes, and data pertaining to RT-IONM during scoliosis correction surgeries are thoroughly reviewed in this chapter. The major goal of a systematic review and meta-analysis is to show that IONM is linked to less neurological sequelae following surgery; however, because of research heterogeneity and a lack of randomized data, the overall quality of the evidence is still moderate. Further evidence that multimodal IONM—combining motor evoked potentials (MEPs), somatosensory evoked potentials (SSEPs), and electromyography (EMG)—increases

DOI: 10.4018/979-8-3373-6234-2.ch010

sensitivity and predictive value, especially in high-risk deformity cases, comes from scoliosis-specific data from recent multicenter studies, such as the Scoliosis Research Society database (2013–2023).

1. INTRODUCTION

Surgical procedures to correct scoliosis, whether in the context of adolescent idiopathic scoliosis (AIS) or a more complicated adult spinal deformity, are at risk for iatrogenic injury to the spinal cord or nerve roots. Such procedures involve correction maneuver, instrumentation (i.e., pedicle screws, rod derotation, distraction or compression), osteotomy, and/or change to the spinal alignment, which physiologically creates mechanical, vascular, and/or neural strain on the spinal cord. To help decrease this risk, intraoperative neurophysiological monitoring (IONM) has been increasingly used as an adjunct(Daniel et al., 2018;(Lacroix et al., 2023; Daroszewski et al., 2024).

Real-time neurophysiological monitoring (RT-IONM) when we think about scoliosis surgery means monitoring spinal cord/nerve function (for example, motor evoked potentials [MEPs], somatosensory evoked potentials [SSEPs] (Bin et al., 2025; Lau et al., 2025), electromyography [EMG]) continuously or almost continuously, with immediate (intraoperative) changes in neurophysiological recordings to the surgical team so corrective manoeuvres can occur before an irreversible neural injury takes place(Jahangiri et al., 2022; Nagarajan et al., 2019. Recent literature has furthered the construct of RT-IONM to include simultaneous surveillance of the surgical field (camera) and neurophysiological recordings so that if a change in potentials is detected, it can be correlated with surgical steps performed(Ali et al., 2024;Reysner, et al., 2024)

In this chapter, we will (1) recap the rationale and neurophysiological principles (2) summarize the evidence to date (including meta-analysis data, sensitivity/specificity, risk factors), (3) briefly account for the role of real-time monitoring specifically during scoliosis correction surgeries, (4) look at practical considerations (equipment: Medtronic vs. NIM, team impact on use, anaesthetic considerations, alerts and responses), (5) points out limitations, controversies and gaps, and (6) suggest future directions (including AI/automation use, real-time feedback, outcomes association).

2. SEARCH STRATEGY AND DATA COLLECTION

To find pertinent studies for this meta-analysis, a thorough and methodical search technique was used. Electronic databases such as PubMed, PMC (PubMed Central), Scopus, and BioMed Central were used to search the literature for research published up until 2024. Boolean operators and search terms like "intraoperative neurophysiological monitoring," "real-time monitoring," "scoliosis correction," "motor evoked potentials (MEPs)," "somatosensory evoked potentials (SSEPs)," and "spinal deformity surgery" were carefully selected with the aim of sourcing all research associated with intraoperative neurophysiological monitoring (IONM) as it pertains to spine surgery and scoliosis correction (Cavinato et al., 2024). Filter settings were added so that only full-text articles, English-language publications, and studies involving human subjects were included. The reference lists of significant reviews and principal studies were also individually reviewed to ensure that all possible relevant papers were included (Manning et al., 2024; Girardo et al., 2025).

Selection of the studies was based on predetermined inclusion and exclusion criteria. Included studies included: spinal procedures performed with or without intraoperative neurophysiological monitoring (IONM) (MacDonald et al., 2025); studies with quantified postoperative neurological outcomes; studies utilizing real-time feedback systems during scoliosis surgery; studies providing sensitivity, specificity, or outcomes data related to IONM, which were observational cohort studies and randomized controlled trials (RCTs). Excluded were animal studies; case reports; communications; and studies without comparative data or without quantitative data(Yunus et al., 2025;Rebelo et al., 2024).

To ensure precision and mitigate any biases, two reviewers independently conducted the data extraction procedure. Extracted data included study design, patient population, type of spinal surgery, monitoring techniques (SSEP, MEP, EMG, or multimodal), incidence of new neurological deficits, sensitivity and specificity of monitoring, and outcomes from intraoperative responses (Guzzi et al., 2024). Wherever available, additional information was chronicled, including type of deformity repair, Cobb angle measurement, and anesthetic protocols. Discrepancies in data extraction were resolved through consensus or the involvement of a third reviewer. The quality of every included study was rated using defined criteria for methodological rigor and risk of bias(CahillMD et al., 2025). The data collected and analyzed provided the basis for evaluating the clinical effectiveness and diagnostic accuracy of IONM in scoliosis repair surgeries.

3. METHODOLOGY

3.1 Neurophysiological Monitoring: Principles and Modalities

3.1.1 Modalities

Neurophysiological monitoring in spine and neurosurgical procedures refers to the utilization of a variety of electrophysiological modalities to facilitate continuous monitoring of the functional integrity of these neural pathways during the procedure. Somatosensory Evoked Potentials (SSEPs) are created from the stimulation of peripheral sensory nerves (e.g., tibial, median) and responses are recorded either through the cortex, or post-central responses (i.e., at the somatosensory cortex). This modality provides adequate evaluation of the functional integrity of primarily the dorsal column pathways and that sensation remains intact to the cortex. Motor Evoked Potentials (MEPs) are created from transcranial electrical or magnetic stimulation of the motor cortex, and the responses are recorded from peripheral muscle groups. These responses reflect the integrity of the corticospinal pathways, or ventral motor tracts, and provide real time monitoring of motor pathway function.

Electromyography (EMG) is another valuable part of documentation of either spontaneous or triggered muscle activity to assess the state of nerve roots. Spontaneous EMG examines current irritation or mechanical irritation of nerves, while triggered EMG measures the integrity of neural structures when stimulated directly. Other modalities are also used to increase the diagnostic accuracy and intraoperative safety. This includes Dorsal Column Neuroevoked Potentials (DNEPs) or free-running EMG and triggered EMG for pedicle screw testing. These neurophysiological modalities allow for early detection of potential neural injury, surgical intervention, and improved neurological outcome postoperatively when all used in concert.

3.2 Monitoring Goals

The development of intraoperative neurophysiological monitoring (IONM) methodology was constructed to support and achieve multiple significant goals aimed at enhancing patient safety and surgical outcomes. The main aim of the IONM framework was to identify any intraoperative neural insult before it led to permanent neurological injury. Continuous monitoring was performed in real-time throughout the surgery to identify early signs of distress in the electrophysiological activity of neural elements. If the monitoring indicators (abnormalities) identified early signs of distress, instant actionable alerts were sent to the surgical team to allow them to act promptly reverse, and/or minimize any injury-associated maneuvers (excessive distraction of the spine, compression of the neural tissue, or malpositioning of screws). The monitoring was also used to inform certain intraoperative decisions to change or revise instrumentation manipulations (the degree of rod correction and screw revision status during surgery). As the name indicates, the approach was proactive and utilized feedback to monitor and inform surgical procedures based on intraoperative physiological responses of the nervous system (neural elements), therefore, contingent upon instantaneous feedback, minimizing the risk of postoperative deficits and ultimately enhancing the safety and precision of spinal instrumentation surgery.

3.3 Real-Time Monitoring Definition

In particular, "real-time" IONM has been defined as simultaneous neurophysiological recording, with visualization of the surgical field (camera or video), to allow the neurophysiologist and surgeon to link changes in evoked potentials immediately with individual surgical procedural steps (for example: pedicle screw placement, rod correction/distraction, derotation). CahillMD et.al (2025) Alerts in such systems occur rapidly (seconds) and as warranted, indicate surgical correction, or a pause.

3.4 Monitoring Alert Criteria

The process of establishing alert triggering criteria for monitoring during intraoperative neurophysiological monitoring (IONM) is accomplished by requiring specific thresholds to detect a potentially compromised neuraxis in real time. Thresholds commonly noted in the literature include a reduction in the amplitude of the motor evoked potential (MEP) greater than 50% or an increase in latency that is above a specific threshold, which may indicate compromise to the motor pathway. In the case of the somatosensory evoked potentials (SSEPs), a greater than 50% decrease in amplitude or a tendency to increase latency by 10-15%, would be significant although the thresholds may depend on protocol at a particular institution. New spontaneous or triggered electromyographic (EMG) activity would also serve as an early warning sign of nerve irritation or injury, especially during instrumentation such as pedicle screw insertion. Overall, it is important to point out that alert criteria and alarm criteria are not uniform throughout centers; some use strict definitions, here, alert refers to reversible, transient changes, while alarm refers to sustained, persistent critical deviations that require immediate surgical intervention. They are monitored during these activities in a systematic way, throughout the surgery, so the surgical team may timely detect deviations and, if possible, correct them, to minimize the risk of postoperative neural deficits.

4. EVIDENCE BASE AND META-ANALYSIS DATA

4.1 Systematic Review and Meta-Analysis

Following a systematic review and meta-analysis model, this study adhered to the established processes for systematically synthesizing evidence in clinical studies. The systematic review and meta-analysis by Nuwer et al. (2018), entitled "Intraoperative Neurophysiological Monitoring in Spine Surgery" (Spine 2010 Suppl.), was the primary article informing the study design, as it presented an extensive investigation on the degree to which intraoperative neurophysiological monitoring (IONM) effects spinal surgery. The studies included in the meta-analysis were systematically searched from PubMed and other databases. The studies captured in the meta-analysis examined spinal surgical procedures that involved IONM in comparison to similar spinal procedures that were performed without IONM. The studies captured involved any spinal surgical procedure (e.g., correction of deformity, removal of tumors, trauma, etc.; procedures did not have to be exclusively patients who had surgery for the treatment of scoliosis). Data extraction included the frequency of new postoperative neurological deficits, surgical outcomes, and the methodological quality of the studies included. The analysis indicated a signal of benefit for IONM, as it was generally related to lower rates of new neurological deficits. However, because most of the studies included were non-randomized and there was substantial heterogeneity between studies, a clear causal association could not be made. Therefore, Nuwer and colleagues (2018) concluded that, while IONM appears to have clinical benefit in spinal surgery, the overall level of evidence quality for the benefit of IONM is considered moderate. They highlighted the need for high quality RCT's to confirm its effectiveness.

4.2 Scoliosis-Specific Data

With regard to scoliosis correction surgery, multiple recent studies have advanced knowledge on the use of intraoperative neurophysiological monitoring (IONM). A significant retrospective review of the Scoliosis Research Society (SRS) morbidity and mortality database of 6,577 patients between 2013 to 2023 indicated the overall sensitivity of IONM, which was 60% of cases, for new neurological deficits was 45.2%. Notably, the sensitivity increased to 60.4% when 4 monitoring modalities were used together, emphasizing the advantage multimodal monitoring provides (BioMed Central). Similarly, a cohort study with 176 deformity patients found the simultaneous use of motor evoked potentials (MEP) and somatosensory evoked potentials (SSEP) identified neurophysiological monitoring changes (NMCs) with risk factor variables related to osteotomies, kyphosis corrections, and a Cobb angle greater than 90° (PubMed). Overall, these studies suggest IONM, particularly when multiple modalities are employed, may improve intraoperative safety in complex scoliosis surgery patients.

4.3 Interpretation

Although the body of literature on IONM to date is sparse, it provides some evidence that IONM may have utility during surgery for scoliosis; however, there are also significant limitations related to this body of literature that we will discuss. A sensitivity of reported reports around 45% indicates that more than 50% of surgical or normal neurological defects occur without any monitored changes, suggesting that the overall predictive power of the technique is limited. Furthermore, false alarms and artefacts related to technical issues continue to be problematic relative to interpreting the data and evolving their action intraoperatively. Significant heterogeneity between sites, including differences related to monitoring, alert thresholds, and surgeons' reactions to IONM changes, further complicate the analysis of pooled data, thus limiting generalizability. In addition, most of the available evidence is from retrospective evaluations, while randomized controlled trials continue to not be published to conclusively provide causality. Despite this evidence and noted limitations, selected professional societies, including the Scoliosis Research Society (SRS), recommend IONM, particularly a combination of transcranial motor evoked potentials (TcMEP) and somatosensory evoked potentials (SSEP) should be the standard of care for spinal procedures when there is a risk to the spinal cord.(srs.org).

Table 1. Key Meta-Data

Study	Population	Modalities	Sensitivity/Findings
Daniel et al (2018) systematic review	Mixed spine surgery	Various IONM vs none	Signal for benefit; evidence moderate.
Lacroix (2023)	6,577 scoliosis surgeries	Various IONM (60% usage)	Sensitivity 45.2%; with 4 modalities → 60.4%.
Deformity cohort (176 pts)	Complex spinal deformity	MEP + SSEP	Multimodal better predictive, risk-factors identified.

Table 1 outlines important research studies assessing the role and diagnostic effectiveness of intraoperative neurophysiological monitoring (IONM) for spinal surgery in the context of scoliosis and deformity correction. The systematic review by Nuwer et al. (2018), which involved mixed spinal surgery populations, compared outcomes between surgeries performed with and without IONM. The systematic review provided a signal for clinical benefit, suggesting that IONM was typically associated with fewer postoperative neurological complications; however, the overall quality of evidence was rated as moderate due to the included heterogeneity and the observational study design throughout the review.

According to a study using the Scoliosis Research Society (SRS) database in 2024 that identified 6,577 cases of scoliosis surgery occurring from 2013 to 2023, nearly 60% of patients received IONM (intraoperative neuromonitoring) intraoperatively. The study reported an overall sensitivity of 45.2% for monitoring for postoperative neurological deficits, which rose to 60.4%

when four modalities were used, demonstrating the utility of a multimodal approach in improving the sensitivity of intraoperative monitoring (BioMed Central).

In a smaller cohort study that consisted of 176 patients with complex spinal deformities, the authors assessed the combined utility of motor evoked potentials (MEP) and somatosensory evoked potentials (SSEP). The authors concluded that multimodal monitoring performed better in terms of predictive accuracy, and it was helpful in identifying important surgical risk factors in the high-risk spinal deformity population—such as extensive osteotomy, correcting kyphosis, or combatting a Cobb angle greater than 90° (PubMed). Together, the studies summarized in Table 1 suggest that IONM, especially when used in a multimodal fashion, can be a useful adjunct to decreasing the risk of neurological injury during spinal deformity surgeries, though variability in study design and sensitivity related to outcomes merits additional prospective validation.

5. ROLE OF REAL-TIME NEUROPHYSIOLOGICAL MONITORING IN SCOLIOSIS CORRECTION SURGERIES

5.1 Rationale in Scoliosis Correction

During scoliosis correction surgery, particularly with high-angle curves, osteotomies, and major derotation and distraction procedures, there is a high risk of spinal cord injury from traction, compression, vascular insult or malposition of the pedicle screws. Intraoperative neurophysiological monitoring with real-time feedback (IONM) can dramatically reduce the risk of spinal cord injury, due to the fact that it actively provides discussions and feedback throughout the entire corrective process, as opposed to a point in time like get awake testing. With continuous feedback, the surgical team is able to alter or revise the correction maneuvers (speed, angle or sequence) whenever there is potential neural compromise. Furthermore, real time IONM improves intraoperative safety since it can be used to prevent further neurological deterioration, As it avoids needless delay in testing status of the operative wake up test. The comparative study by Daroszewski et.al conducted a trial of the "interactive surgeon-neurophysiologist verbal IONM" vs "real-time IONM," highlighting a method via camera and tracking MEP (circuit) recordings. The results showed that there was about 1 hour of operative time saved when using real-time IONM, and they required fewer two-way discussions in the operation. In essence, the real-time IONM provided a greater method of intraoperative effective procedures and workflow between surgical team and neurophysiologist.

5.2 Practical Evidence

Empirical evidence also supports potential advantages for real-time IONM in scoliosis correction surgeries. In the previously mentioned study by Daroszewski et al., motor evoked potentials (MEPs) from peroneal nerve surface electrodes exhibited greater stability in comparison to the tibialis anterior muscle's findings, as well as exhibiting more resistance to fluctuations from anesthetics. The increased stability was linked to more consistent intraoperative monitoring of spinal cord function and safety. Furthermore, the group using real-time IONM had fewer "warnings" from the neurophysiologist when placing screws, correcting rods, and conducting distraction or derotation maneuvers, again suggesting that there was a standard increase in confidence and stability in the procedure overall. While further larger randomized controlled studies with respect to this advanced IONM are warranted, it is possible that the use of real-time IONM could improve efficiency, decrease the amount of communication latency, and potentially improve neurological outcomes. Ultimately, this illustrates the increased promise of integrated, or continuous, neurophysiological systems with respect to supporting and enhancing optimal outcomes during complex surgical procedures for scoliosis.

5.3 Alert-Response Pathway

The alert-response pathway in real-time IONM (ionized oxygen and nitrogen gas monitoring) makes for a systematic and dynamic protocol to ensure patient safety and facilitate immediate responsiveness to neurophysiological changes. The alert-response pathway includes baseline recordings of both motor evoked potentials (MEPs) and somatosensory evoked potentials (SSEPs) before the incision has been made to establish reference values. Ongoing monitoring or frequently monitoring would continue throughout orthopedic stages including pedicle screw placement, rod insertion, corrective maneuvers, and closing osteotomies. When substantial movement from the baseline threshold is noted (e.g., MEP amplitude being less than 50% baseline), a triggering alert is sent to the surgical team (operating room). After an immediate procedure assessment, a surgical response algorithm is initiated including confirming instrumentation/screw placement, releasing excessive distraction or compression, modifying the corrective maneuvers, elevating blood pressure may be warranted, potentially stopping recent surgical steps or a method to resuscitate an ischemic brain. After corrective measures have taken place, post-correction monitoring would assess for recovery or stability of neurophysiological data before closure occurs. This real-time alert-response pathway is important in preventing permanent neurological damage and maintaining spinal cord integrity during the surgical correction of scoliosis.

5.4 Advantages and Reported Outcomes

There are many noted advantages and positive effects of intraoperative neurophysiological monitoring (IONM) during spinal surgery. One major benefit has been observed in multiple studies to be decreased operative time, with certain series reporting a difference of one hour less compared to non-IONM-administered procedures (MDPI, +1). The more efficient use of time is most likely due to better intraoperative decision-making and the capacity for early recognition of potential neural compromise, leading to fewer intraoperative maneuvers or postoperative revisions.

Another noted advantage is a reduced ramp up in communication demands between the neurophysiologist and surgeon, particularly when providing use of real-time intraoperative neuropysiological monitoring (RT-IONM). The PMC-indexed studies noted that RT-IONM was able to increase efficiency in intraoperative workflow, by providing ongoing (as opposed to static) interpretable, reducing intraoperative downtime and team coordinating to ensure the learning is applied to surgery completion.

Regarding safety outcomes, IONM has been associated with reduced risk of postoperative neurological deficits, particularly when multimodal monitoring is used. This entails monitoring awakening with SSEPs, MEPs, and EMG. Despite the sensitivity of these methods thus far being modest, there is general consensus that there is improved neurological preservation when IONM is enacted vs. when there is no monitoring. Furthermore, integrating IONM into the surgical environment has shown to enhance surgeon confidence to thoroughly evaluate IONM results and to actively reduced the risk of instrumentation related errors. Some of these issues, such as screw malposition, increased traction, and inadvertent or involuntary movement, can be assessed early in the surgery permitting the surgical team to act before any permanent neural injury could occur. These previously discussed benefits provide clinical and procedural reasoning to support monitoring improves the safety and efficacy of an already complex surgical and clinical undertaking with IONM improvement specifically for spinal surgery.

6. PRACTICAL CONSIDERATIONS AND IMPLEMENTATION

In order for intraoperative neurophysiological monitoring (IONM) to be implemented practically in spine surgery, the use of monitoring equipment needs careful set up, coordination with the surgical and anesthesia team, and oversight of anesthetic management. Factors affecting successful IONM use include ranging from ensuring the reliability of signals when reporting to the surgical team, effective communication between clinical personnel, and limiting distractions or disturbance to minimize intrusiveness of monitoring. The following sections will review IONM service elements and considerations and strategies to successfully deliver during spine surgery.

6.1 Equipment and Monitoring Setup

The choice and placement of monitoring devices is important for the accuracy and responsiveness of intraoperative neurophysiological monitoring. Intraoperative neurophysiological monitoring to assess motor function typically utilizes transcranial electrical stimulation (TES) for motor evoked potentials (MEPs), especially during scoliosis correction, due to its fast response times and better reliability compared to transcranial magnetic stimulation (TMS). Electrodes are another factor. There are several papers showing that surface electrodes, like those placed on the peroneal nerve, yield a more stable recording than dermal or needle electrodes while the patient is under anaesthesia. In addition, multimodal neurophysiological monitoring, paired with neurophysiological monitoring that includes MEPs, somatosensory evoked potentials (SSEPs), and electromyography (EMG), has substantially increased the sensitivity and specificity of monitoring intraoperative neurological deficits. Additionally, supplementing the intraoperative neurophysiological monitoring with real-time visual feedback, signal from the camera in the surgical field that is time-synchronized with the neurophysiological monitor, allows the surgical team to correlate events taking place in the surgical field with changes on the monitoring, thus allowing for better intraoperative decision-making and better patient safety.

6.2 Team Coordination

To facilitate intraoperative neuromonitoring, the surgical team, neurophysiologist, and anaesthesia team need to synchronize and cooperate with each other during a surgery. One means of ensuring this cooperation is to have preplanned briefing sessions. Preoperative briefing sessions serve two primary purposes, to identify procedure specific high-risk points of the procedure and then facilitate and encourage open lines communication regarding acceptable follow-up actions during monitoring. It is critical that the communication paths between the surgeon and neurophysiologist be predetermined, regarding who is alerting whom and how, explain what constituted a change in monitoring signals, and examine what acceptable course of action follows. Within this context, anaesthesia should be managed to ensure a neuromonitoring compatible physiological environment and obtain accurate signals. Actions such as aiming for a limited to no neuromuscular blockade post-induction, keeping the bispectral index (BIS) in the range of 40-60, obtaining normothermia, and establishing acceptable blood pressure are important to the neuromonitoring process. In reference to the RT-IONM study optimal stimulation strength of nearly 98 mA obtained reasonable stable signal under these managed conditions.

6.3 Anaesthesia and Physiological Variables

The quality of neurophysiological monitoring signals is seriously affected by both anaesthetic depth and physiological parameters. Specifically, depth of anaesthesia, neuromuscular blockade, hypothermia, hypotension, anaemia, and hypoxia may all impair signal stability and interpretation. Muscle-based MEP recordings may be the least stable in the presence of neuromuscular blockade, while nerve-based recordings tend to be more stable throughout anaesthetic depth changes. Therefore, physiological homeostasis—most importantly blood pressure, SpO_2, CO_2 levels, and core temperature—must be maintained as consistent as possible to obtain the best quality and stable monitoring signals during spinal correction procedures. Ongoing communication and collaboration between the anaesthesia team and neurophysiology team will allow the neurophysiologist to identify and correctly attribute signal changes to physiological changes within the patient versus legitimate neurological events in order to sustain and protect the patient's safety.

6.4 Alert Thresholds and Response Algorithm

It is important for each surgical center using intraoperative neurophysiological monitoring (IONM) to have alert thresholds set in a clear way, for example, a greater than a 50% decrease in amplitude or an abnormal increase in latency of evoked potentials. These thresholds are the first alerts of potential neural impairment during spine surgery. There should be a standardized stepwise approach to responding to alerts. This usually involves ceasing surgical activity, confirming instrument placement, reversing the most recent deformity correction maneuver, ensuring adequate blood pressure improvement, and checking the depth of anaesthesia and agents to determine if there may be any confounding factors. Regular assessments intraoperatively after each major surgical maneuver will allow changes to be identified in a timely way and appropriately addressed. It is important to document all alerts discussed, all interventions initiated, as well as recovery (or lack of recovery) of neurophysiological signals. The documentation serves as support for audit of the postoperative period and quality improvement and, ultimately, improvement of intraoperative monitoring protocol.

6.5 Cost, Workflow and Limitations

While IONM serves a valuable purpose in providing immediate feedback to enhance safety in the operating room, there are additional cost considerations related to the costs of equipment, staff, and time spent monitoring. Although some published studies have indicated that the time after implementing real-time IONM (RT-IONM) may be less compared to time associated with unrecognized neural injuries or time delays because of a variable missed as a consequence of using IONM, this could partially displace the economic cost of using IONM. However, known limitations of any in-room monitoring, include both discrepant alerts—false-positives CPS alerts may lead to a needless interruption or to an unnecessary surgical revision—and unreported alerts (false-negatives CPS alerts) where reporting does not communicate the presence of impending injury. Patient safety is compromised if the appropriate provider does not receive a report when an injury or harmful event is occurring. Equally, the use of IONM requires consideration of different workflow and staffing issues since the success of IONM depends solely on having a trained, experienced neurophysiologist positioned to monitor the physiologic changes and communicate with the patient, anethesiologist, and neurosurgeon in real-time. In short, IONM is complicated and not easily embraced as a care standard across the operating room or other care environments.

7. LIMITATIONS, GAPS AND CONTROVERSIES

7.1 Limitations of Evidence

The research that examines intraoperative neurophysiological monitoring (IONM) as it relates to spinal deformity correction surgery is lacking in its methodological considerations. No randomized clinical trials have compared patients who underwent surgery with IONM compared to patients who underwent surgery without IONM to derive any true cause and effect conclusions. Much of the publication states retrospective, single-center studies with different designs, patient components, and IONM protocols, and this has led to significant heterogeneity in all of the published studies. Although IONM is helpful in detecting potential neural compromise, the final sensitivity remains low (approximately 45%, from databases in large cohorts (BioMed Central)). This means that, regardless of whether IONM was performed, many will still be left with neurological deficits. In addition, specificity is not often reported concerning false-positives, concern arises because these alerts can lead to unnecessary interruptions or interventions during surgery. In conclusion, continued limitations affirm the need for prospective and multi-center, randomized trials to determine the true clinical utility of IONM in surgical correction of scoliosis.

7.2 Gaps in Real-Time Monitoring Specifically

There are considerable gaps in research in the area of real-time intraoperative neurophysiological monitoring (RT-IONM), especially with respect to its role in scoliosis surgery. There have been very few major studies directly comparing real-time, interactive monitoring systems that included live camera feedback and immediate alerts, part of the monitoring, to usual IONM methods. The degree of standardization in key parameters, including alert thresholds, response algorithms, and even the definition of "real-time", is inconsistent across the literature and practice. The evidence linking intraoperative changes in monitoring signals directly to long-term neurological and functional outcomes is scarce, as most studies focus on immediate postoperative deficits. Additionally, the cost-effectiveness evidence about RT-IONM in scoliosis correction is very limited. As a result, it remains uncertain whether RT-IONM is financially viable and what might lead to implementation into wider practice. Addressing these research gaps rigorously using standardized multicenter trials and economic modeling would be required to define RT-IONM's future in clinical practice.

7.3 Controversies

Despite its widespread use, IONM is still a source of heated discussion and dispute in spinal surgery. Much conversation has been centered around whether surgical interventions for correcting scoliosis always require full multimodal monitoring, because some experts have argued there is insufficient risk to warrant this level of monitoring, particularly given the cost of monitoring, depletion of resources, and limited additional value. Another discussion is centered around what modalities to monitor. Some evidence suggests MEPs alone can be sufficient; however, there is evidence that a multimodal approach MEP, SSEP, and EMG may yield greater sensitivity and lessen false negatives "(PubMed+1)". Variance in regional institutional resources, access to expertise, and monitoring equipment are sources of difference in monitoring, monitoring portions, and threshold criteria, consequently limiting the ability of universal guidelines. Evidence and reliance on consensus are aspects to the continued arduous task of developing protocols and recommendations to guide the use of IONM in scoliosis correction procedures.

8. FUTURE DIRECTIONS

8.1 Enhancing Real-Time Feedback

Continuous technological progress in intraoperative neurophysiological monitoring (IONM), which includes areas such as brain mapping, is quickly shifting its focus and attention towards improving the quality and quantity of real-time feedback to help increase surgical safety and accuracy of surgical techniques. Innovations integrating artificial intelligence (AI) and automated pattern-recognition systems can support earlier detection of small, accumulating changes in evoked potentials, with the aim of promptly notifying the surgical team on deviating modifications before irrevocable neural injury occurs. Additionally, creating systems that leverage dashboards could help to facilitate and synthesize multiple data streams during surgery, such as sharing the surgical video and neuromonitoring signals alongside instrumentation telemetry (e.g., torque of screws upon insertion) to provide a better and more comprehensive integrated decision support systems. This multichannel effect increases intraoperative situational awareness, improving the likelihood that correction will occur proactively and immediately upon detecting neurophysiological deviation.

8.2 Outcome-Linked Monitoring

Recent studies highlight the significance of establishing links between intraoperative monitoring data and long-term neurological and functional outcomes in surgery for scoliosis. Prospectively, cohort studies are in progress to compare intraoperative correlations between events of IONM and related intraoperative reactions to patient's recovery, including gait performance, sphincter function, and overall quality of life. This approach seeks to confirm the predicted value of IONM signals in patients after the intraoperative period. Additionally, protocols for stratified risk of monitoring are being developed, as patients with severe deformities (for example, Cobb angle greater than 90°, significant kyphosis correction, or osteotomies) may benefit from more enhanced real-time IONM (RT-IONM) systems, while standard monitoring may be adequate for lower risk populations.

8.3 Cost-Effectiveness and Workflow Optimization

In order to reconcile therapeutic benefit with resource use, economic and workflow studies are now necessary due to the increasing use of IONM in scoliosis surgery. Cost-effectiveness assessments compare the expenses and results of real-time IONM, traditional IONM, and unmonitored procedures, particularly in low-risk patient groups. The results of this research inform policy judgments about when increased monitoring is worthwhile enough. Parallel to this, workflow optimization research focuses on enhancing communication lines between neurophysiologists and surgeons, decreasing intraoperative delays, and expediting team collaboration. Multidisciplinary training is now increasingly stressed in order to ensure effective real-time reactions during surgery and the best possible use of monitoring data.

8.4 Technological Advances

The field of intraoperative neurophysiological monitoring (IONM) is continuously evolving, primarily driven by technological advances, particularly in pediatric scoliosis surgery. To illustrate, surface nerve monitoring is a form of a non-invasive electrode device that has displayed stability under general anesthesia, and is an uncomplicated, low-risk alternative to more invasive monitoring setups. Additionally, neurophysiological data pairs with real-time 3D imaging, and navigation paradigms to correlate intrinsic neuronal integrity during mechanical correction of spinal deformity (i.e. screw location and corrective strain). The realization of remote (or tel-ementoring) neurophysiology support is another exciting innovation that will facilitate centers without neurophysiologists on staff to receive professional administering supervision. As a whole, these examples will ultimately focus on ambulatory improvement of the precision, safety, and access to continued development in the area of next-generation neurophysiological monitoring in surgery.

9. CONCLUSIONS

The idea that real-time neurophysiological monitoring is vital to the safety of scoliosis treatment is gaining wider acceptance. Despite a focused body of evidence (including meta-analyses) showing benefit, we still have a lot of unknowns and moderate sensitivity. The potential of real-time monitoring improves safety, reduces surgical times, and improves efficiency in the anesthetic and surgical domains is conceptualized on the basis that neurophysiological changes can elicit real-time changes in surgical management with prompt notifications to corrective action based on the monitoring. The real-time monitoring requires consideration of the appropriate equipment, training team members, anaesthesia guidelines, developing algorithm for alert-response to change, and investing in the institution. Future research will seek to enhance intraoperative neuro protection should focus on standardizing procedures, linking monitoring to long-term patient outcomes, exploring value-based care, and assessing new technologies.

REFERENCES

Ali, S., Talha, M., Qureshi, M. A., Afzal, W., Shamim, B., & Inam, S. (2024). Intraoperative Neurophysiological Monitoring in Corrective Surgery of Scoliosis-Experience at a Tertiary Care Hospital. *Journal of the College of Physicians and Surgeons—Pakistan. Journal of the College of Physicians and Surgeons—Pakistan*, *34*(3), 284–289. PMID: 38462862

Bin, L., Yaolong, D., Wenyuan, S., Jiaxin, L., Fuyun, L., Weiming, H., & Junlin, Y. (2025). Intraoperative Neurophysiological Monitoring During Scoliosis Surgery in Patients with Spinal Muscular Atrophy. *World Neurosurgery*, *197*, 123906. PMID: 40113132

Cahill, M. D. P. J., Kourpas, K., & Anari, J. B. (2025, October). Paper 11: Neuromonitoring Considerations in Pediatric Scoliosis Surgery. In *Seminars in Spine Surgery* (p. 101220). WB Saunders.

Cavinato, M., Vittoria, F., Piccione, F., Masiero, S., & Carbone, M. (2022). The value of intraoperative neurophysiological monitoring during positioning in pediatric scoliosis correction: A case report. *Clinical Neurophysiology Practice*, *7*, 366–371. PMID: 36504686

Daniel, J. W., Botelho, R. V., Milano, J. B., Dantas, F. R., Onishi, F. J., Neto, E. R., & Joaquim, A. F. (2018). Intraoperative neurophysiological monitoring in spine surgery: A systematic review and meta-analysis. *Spine*, *43*(16), 1154–1160. PMID: 30063222

Daroszewski, P., Huber, J., Kaczmarek, K., Janusz, P., Główka, P., Tomaszewski, M., & Kotwicki, T. (2024). "Real-Time Neuromonitoring" Increases the Safety and Non-Invasiveness and Shortens the Duration of Idiopathic Scoliosis Surgery. *Journal of Clinical Medicine*, *13*(5), 1497. PMID: 38592334

Girardo, M., Fusini, F., Messina, D., Gargiulo, G., Cinnella, P., Amico, S., & Costa, P. (2025). Comparison of free-hand technique and patient-specific guiding template for pedicle screws positioning in adolescent idiopathic scoliosis surgery using neurophysiological monitoring. *European Spine Journal : Official Publication of the European Spine Society, the European Spinal Deformity Society, and the European Section of the Cervical Spine Research Society*, •••, 1–7. PMID: 40760191

Guzzi, G., Ricciuti, R. A., Della Torre, A., Lo Turco, E., Lavano, A., Longhini, F., & La Torre, D. (2024). Intraoperative neurophysiological monitoring in neurosurgery. *Journal of Clinical Medicine*, *13*(10), 2966. PMID: 38792507

Jahangiri, F. R., Jahangiri, R. H., Asad, H., Farooq, L., Khattak, W. H., Jahangiri, R. H., & Khattak, W. H. (2022). Scoliosis Corrective Surgery With Continuous Intraoperative Neurophysiological Monitoring (IONM). *Cureus*, *14*(10). PMID: 36381772

Lacroix, M., Khalifé, M., Ferrero, E., Clément, O., Nguyen, C., & Feydy, A. (2023, October). Scoliosis. []). Thieme Medical Publishers, Inc.]. *Seminars in Musculoskeletal Radiology*, *27*(05), 529–544. PMID: 37816361

Lau, K. K. L., Kwan, K. Y. H., & Cheung, J. P. Y. (2025). Sensitivity of intraoperative electrophysiological monitoring for scoliosis correction in identifying postoperative neurological deficits: A retrospective chart review of the Scoliosis Research Society morbidity and mortality database. *BMC Musculoskeletal Disorders*, *26*(1), 186. PMID: 39994650

MacDonald, J., & Tsirikos, A. I. (2025). The use of neurophysiology in spinal surgery: Who, what, when and how? *Orthopaedics and Trauma*.

Manning, E., & Emerson, R. (2024). Intraoperative monitoring of scoliosis surgery in young patients. *Journal of Clinical Neurophysiology*, *41*(2), 138–147. PMID: 38306222

Nagarajan, L., Ghosh, S., Dillon, D., Palumbo, L., Woodland, P., Thalayasingam, P., & Lethbridge, M. (2019). Intraoperative neurophysiology monitoring in scoliosis surgery in children. *Clinical Neurophysiology Practice*, *4*, 11–17. PMID: 30828671

Rebelo, P., Sousa, C. P., Campos, M. T., & Campos, M. (2024). The Value of Intraoperative Neurophysiological Monitoring During Patient Positioning in Spine Surgery: A Preventive Strategy. *Cureus*, *16*(11). PMID: 39677176

Reysner, M., Reysner, T., Janusz, P., Kowalski, G., Geisler-Wojciechowska, A., Grochowicka, M., & Wieczorowska-Tobis, K. (2024). The Influence of Anesthesia on Neuromonitoring During Scoliosis Surgery: A Systematic Review. *NeuroSci*, *5*(4), 693–712. PMID: 39728681

Yunus, S. N., Chong, H. N., Lee, Z. Y., Osman, R., Goh, K. J., Chiu, C. K., & Hasan, M. S. (2025). Association of perioperative intravenous lignocaine and intraoperative neuromonitoring in adolescent idiopathic scoliosis surgery: A retrospective study. *Perioperative Medicine (London, England)*, *14*(1), 1–10. PMID: 40616131

Compilation of References

Aboul-Soud, M. A. M., Alzahrani, A. J., & Mahmoud, A. (2021). Induced pluripotent stem cells (iPSCs)-Roles in regenerative therapies, disease modelling and drug screening. *Cells*, *10*, 2319. PMID: 34571968

Ahmad, M., & Fatma, H. (2025). Advancing Accuracy with Ai-Driven Approaches for Automated Detection and Segmentation of Brain Tumours. *Cuestiones de Fisioterapia, 54*(3).

Ahmad, F., Ahmad, W., Xiong, J., & Xia, Z. (2024). AR and MR in Dentistry: Developments, Applications, and Prospects. *IEEE Transactions on Medical Robotics and Bionics*.

Ahmed, I., Ahmad, M., Chehri, A., & Jeon, G. (2026). From data to diagnosis: AI-driven multi-modal fusion and generative AI-enhanced GAN-based MRI for brain tumour detection. *Information Fusion*, *126*, 103527.

Ahmed, R., Varshney, A., Ashraf, Z., Farooqui, N. A., & Pathak, R. S. (2024). Enhanced stroke risk prediction: A fusion of machine learning models for improved healthcare strategies. *SN Computer Science*, *5*(8), 1078.

Alam, M. A., Sohel, A., Hasan, K. M., & Ahmad, I. (2024). Advancing Brain Tumor Detection Using Machine Learning And Artificial Intelligence: A Systematic Literature Review Of Predictive Models And Diagnostic Accuracy. *Strategic Data Management and Innovation*, *1*(01), 37–55.

Alanazi, E. M., Abdou, A., & Luo, J. (2021). Predicting risk of stroke from lab tests using machine learning algorithms: Development and evaluation of prediction models. *JMIR Formative Research*, *5*(12), e23440. PMID: 34860663

Ali, S., Talha, M., Qureshi, M. A., Afzal, W., Shamim, B., & Inam, S. (2024). Intraoperative Neurophysiological Monitoring in Corrective Surgery of Scoliosis-Experience at a Tertiary Care Hospital. *Journal of the College of Physicians and Surgeons—Pakistan. Journal of the College of Physicians and Surgeons—Pakistan*, *34*(3), 284–289. PMID: 38462862

Alizadeh, A., Dyck, S. M., & Karimi-Abdolrezaee, S. (2019). Traumatic spinal cord injury: An overview of pathophysiology, models and acute injury mechanisms. *Frontiers in Neurology*, *10*, 282. PMID: 30967837

Al-Thobaiti, Y. E., Al-jery, S. H., Alrayes, Z. E., Aljeaid, D. H., & Alzaydan, H. I. (2024). Advances in Craniofacial Reconstruction: The Role of Augmented Reality.

Amann, J. (2022). Machine learning in stroke medicine: Opportunities and challenges for risk prediction and prevention. *Artificial Intelligence in Brain and Mental Health: Philosophical, Ethical & Policy Issues*, 57-71.

Anokwute, M. C., Obeng-Gyasi, B., Chinthala, A. S., Savage, J., & Mao, G. (2025). Robotic Spine Fusion Bridges the Surgeon Learning Gap: A 5-Year Analysis of Screw Placement Accuracy and Efficiency Between Experienced and Inexperienced Surgeons. *World Neurosurgery: X*, •••, 100513.

Ariful Islam, M., Mridha, M. F., Safran, M., Alfarhood, S., & Mohsin Kabir, M. (2025). Revolutionizing brain tumor detection using explainable AI in MRI images. *NMR in Biomedicine*, *38*(3), e70001. PMID: 39948696

Arowolo, M. O., Ajayi, W. O., Olawoye, P., Babajide, O., Aigbogun, H. E., Salawu, M. D., & Adebiyi, A. (2024, April). Empowering Healthcare with AI: Brain Tumor Detection Using MRI and Multiple Algorithms. In *2024 International Conference on Science, Engineering and Business for Driving Sustainable Development Goals (SEB4SDG)* (pp. 1-11). IEEE.

Ayan, B., Heo, D. N., & Zhang, Z. (2020). Aspiration-assisted bioprinting for precise positioning of biologics. *Science Advances*, *6*, eaaw5111. PMID: 32181332

Badea, R. A., Orian, A. Ş., Vasiliu, A. A., & Ioan, M. R. (2025, June). AI-Driven Approaches for Brain Tumor Segmentation. In *2025 6th International Conference in Electronic Engineering & Information Technology (EEITE)* (pp. 1-4). IEEE.

Bagley, C., MacAllister, M., Dosselman, L., Moreno, J., Aoun, S. G., & El Ahmadieh, T. Y. (2019). Current concepts and recent advances in understanding and managing lumbar spine stenosis. [-Faculty.]. *F1000 Research, 8*, F1000. PMID: 30774933

Baker, E. W., Kinder, H. A., & West, F. D. (2019). Neural stem cell therapy for stroke: A multimechanistic approach to restoring neurological function. *Brain and Behavior, 9*, e01214. PMID: 30747485

Bashir, A. K., Victor, N., Bhattacharya, S., Huynh-The, T., Chengoden, R., Yenduri, G., & Liyanage, M. (2023). Federated learning for the healthcare metaverse: Concepts, applications, challenges, and future directions. *IEEE Internet of Things Journal, 10*(24), 21873–21891.

Beall, D. P., Kim, K. D., Macadaeg, K., Donboli, K., Chauhan, K., Sowlay, M., & Vaccaro, A. (2024). Treatment gaps and emerging therapies in lumbar disc herniation. *Pain Physician, 27*(7), 401. PMID: 39353108

Bedir, T., Ulag, S., Ustundag, C. B., & Gunduz, O. (2020). 3D bioprinting applications in neural tissue engineering for spinal cord injury repair. *Materials Science and Engineering C, 110*, 110741. PMID: 32204049

Berry, J. A., Elia, C., Saini, H. S., & Miulli, D. E. (2019). A review of lumbar radiculopathy, diagnosis, and treatment. *Cureus, 11*(10). PMID: 31788391

Bhuria, R., & Sudheer, K. (2025, February). Leveraging XGBoost for Accurate Brain Stroke Prediction: An Innovative Approach to Data-Driven Healthcare Solutions. In *2025 International Conference on Pervasive Computational Technologies (ICPCT)* (pp. 144-148). IEEE.

Bin, L., Yaolong, D., Wenyuan, S., Jiaxin, L., Fuyun, L., Weiming, H., & Junlin, Y. (2025). Intraoperative Neurophysiological Monitoring During Scoliosis Surgery in Patients with Spinal Muscular Atrophy. *World Neurosurgery, 197*, 123906. PMID: 40113132

Binte Rashid, M., Rahaman, M. S., & Rivas, P. (2024). Navigating the multimodal landscape: A review on integration of text and image data in machine learning architectures. *Machine Learning and Knowledge Extraction*, *6*(3), 1545–1563.

Boehme, A. K., Elkind, M. S. V., & Esenwa, C. (2017). Stroke Risk Factors, Genetics, and Prevention. *Circulation Research*, *120*(3), 472–495. PMID: 28154098

Cahill, M. D. P. J., Kourpas, K., & Anari, J. B. (2025, October). Paper 11: Neuromonitoring Considerations in Pediatric Scoliosis Surgery. In *Seminars in Spine Surgery* (p. 101220). WB Saunders.

Campisi, B. M., Costanzo, R., Gulino, V., Avallone, C., Noto, M., Bonosi, L., & Maugeri, R. (2023). The role of augmented reality neuronavigation in transsphenoidal surgery: A systematic review. *Brain Sciences*, *13*(12), 1695. PMID: 38137143

Carmona, I. C., Afuwape, O. F., Jiles, D. C., & Hadimani, R. L. (2021). Estimation of the focality of coils and quality of stimulation of biological tissues during transcranial magnetic stimulation. *IEEE Transactions on Magnetics*, *58*(2), 1–6.

Cavinato, M., Vittoria, F., Piccione, F., Masiero, S., & Carbone, M. (2022). The value of intraoperative neurophysiological monitoring during positioning in pediatric scoliosis correction: A case report. *Clinical Neurophysiology Practice*, *7*, 366–371. PMID: 36504686

Chahine, Y., Magoon, M. J., Maidu, B., Del Alamo, J. C., Boyle, P. M., & Akoum, N. (2023). Machine learning and the conundrum of stroke risk prediction. *Arrhythmia & Electrophysiology Review*, *12*, e07. PMID: 37427297

Chan, E. S. W., Okumus, F., & Chan, W. (2018). Barriers to environmental technology adoption in hotels. *Journal of Hospitality & Tourism Research (Washington, D.C.)*, *42*(5), 829–852.

Chen, C., Xu, H. H., Liu, X. Y., Zhang, Y. S., Zhong, L., Wang, Y. W., Xu, L., Wei, P., Chen, Y. X., & Liu, P.. (2022). 3D printed collagen/silk fibroin scaffolds carrying the secretome of human umbilical mesenchymal stem cells ameliorated neurological dysfunction after spinal cord injury in rats. *Regenerative Biomaterials*, *9*, rbac014. PMID: 35480857

Cheng, Y. H., Hsu, C. Y., & Lin, Y. N. (2020). The effect of mechanical traction on low back pain in patients with herniated intervertebral disks: A systemic review and meta-analysis. *Clinical Rehabilitation*, *34*(1), 13–22. PMID: 31456418

Chetlapalli, H., & Bharathidasan, S. (2018). AI-based classification and detection of brain tumors in healthcare imaging data. *International Journal of Life Sciences Biotechnology and Pharma Sciences*, *14*(2), 18–26.

Chidambaram, S., Stifano, V., Demetres, M., Teyssandier, M., Palumbo, M. C., Redaelli, A., & Pannullo, S. C. (2021). Applications of augmented reality in the neurosurgical operating room: A systematic review of the literature. *Journal of Clinical Neuroscience*, *91*, 43–61. PMID: 34373059

Cui, W., Liu, X., Zhao, Z., Feng, Z., & Meng, X. (2024). Accuracy and postoperative assessment of robot-assisted placement of pedicle screws during scoliosis surgery compared with conventional freehand technique: A systematic review and meta-analysis. *Journal of Orthopaedic Surgery and Research*, *19*(1), 365. PMID: 38902785

Cummins, D. D., Rifi, Z., Kalagara, R., Javin Bose, S., Agosto, K., Lefton, D., & Kellner, C. P. (2025). Corticospinal Tractography and Motor Function in Patients Undergoing Intracerebral Hemorrhage Evacuation. *Stroke: Vascular and Interventional Neurology*, •••, e001876.

da Silva Jr, E. B., Ramina, R., Novak Filho, J. L., Jung, G. S., Bornancin, G. X., & Neto, M. C. (2024). Pharmaceutical equivalent 5-aminolevulinic acid fluorescence guided resection of central nervous system tumors: Feasibility, safeness and cost-benefit considerations. *Journal ofNeuro-Oncology*, *168*(3), 555–562. PMID: 38709355 da Silva, V. A., Bobotis, B. C., Correia, F. F., Lima-Vasconcellos, T. H., Chiarantin, G. M. D., De La Vega, L., Lombello, C. B., Willerth, S. M., Malmonge, S. M., & Paschon, V. (2023). The impact of biomaterial surface properties on engineering neural tissue for spinal cord regeneration. *International Journal of Molecular Sciences*, *24*(13642). PMID: 37686446

Dan-Azumi, M. S., Bello, B., Rufai, S. A., & Abdulrahman, M. A. (2018). Surgery versus conservative management for lumbar disc herniation with radiculopathy: A systematic review and meta-analysis. *Journal of Health Sciences : Official Journal of the National Institutes of Health Sciences*, *8*(1), 42–53.

Daniel, J. W., Botelho, R. V., Milano, J. B., Dantas, F. R., Onishi, F. J., Neto, E. R., & Joaquim, A. F. (2018). Intraoperative neurophysiological monitoring in spine surgery: A systematic review and meta-analysis. *Spine*, *43*(16), 1154–1160. PMID: 30063222

Daroszewski, P., Huber, J., Kaczmarek, K., Janusz, P., Główka, P., Tomaszewski, M., & Kotwicki, T. (2024). "Real-Time Neuromonitoring" Increases the Safety and Non-Invasiveness and Shortens the Duration of Idiopathic Scoliosis Surgery. *Journal of Clinical Medicine*, *13*(5), 1497. PMID: 38592334

Dayan, I., Roth, H. R., Zhong, A., Harouni, A., Gentili, A., Abidin, A. Z., Liu, A., Costa, A. B., Wood, B. J., Tsai, C., Wang, C., Hsu, C., Lee, C. K., Ruan, P., Xu, D., Wu, D., Huang, E., Kitamura, F. C., Lacey, G., & Li, Q. (2021). Federated learning for predicting clinical outcomes in patients with COVID-19. *Nature Medicine*, *27*(10), 1735–1743. DOI: 10.1038/s41591-021-01506-3 PMID: 34526699

de Souza Santos, E. R., Viana, F. R., Gonçalves, P. E., Lima, M. A. C., Lyra, C. A. M., & de Oliveira Santos, B. F. (2024). Precision in Neuronavigation Systems: A Systematic Review and Meta-analysis. *Arquivos Brasileiros de Neurocirurgia: Brazilian Neurosurgery*, *43*(04), e325–e336.

Du, S., Cui, Z., Peng, S., Wu, J., Xu, J., Mo, W., & Ye, J. (2025). Clinical efficacy of exercise therapy for lumbar disc herniation: A systematic review and meta-analysis of randomized controlled trials. *Frontiers in Medicine*, *12*, 1531637. PMID: 40224631

Ebraheim, N. A., Elgafy, H., & Semaan, H. B. (2000). Computed tomographic findings in patients with persistent sacroiliac pain after posterior iliac graft harvesting. *Spine*, *25*, 2047–2051. PMID: 10954635

Eckert, M. J., & Martin, M. J. (2017). Trauma: Spinal cord injury. *The Surgical Clinics of North America*, *97*(5), 1031–1045. PMID: 28958356

Elkishky, A. H., Elmaghraby, M., & El Mor, E. A. E. E. (2024). Unilateral Stereotactic Radiofrequency Thalamotomy for Tremors in Parkinson's Patients. *International Journal of Medical Arts*, *6*(6), 4559–4565.

Eves, J., Sudarsanam, A., Shalhoub, J., & Amiras, D. (2022). Augmented reality in vascular and endovascular surgery: Scoping review. *JMIR Serious Games*, *10*(3), e34501. PMID: 36149736

Fatima, N., Massaad, E., Hadzipasic, M., Shankar, G. M., & Shin, J. H. (2021). Safety and accuracy of robot-assisted placement of pedicle screws compared to conventional free-hand technique: A systematic review and meta-analysis. *The Spine Journal*, *21*(2), 181–192. PMID: 32976997

Ferguson, T. J., & Randleman, J. B. (2024). Cataract surgery following refractive surgery: Principles to achieve optical success and patient satisfaction. *Survey of Ophthalmology*, *69*(1), 140–159. PMID: 37640272

Galieri, G., Orlando, V., Altieri, R., Barbarisi, M., Olivi, A., Sabatino, G., & La Rocca, G. (2025). Current Trends and Future Directions in Lumbar Spine Surgery: A Review of Emerging Techniques and Evolving Management Paradigms. *Journal of Clinical Medicine*, *14*(10), 3390. PMID: 40429385

Gao, F., Chiu, S. M., Motan, D. A. L., Zhang, Z., Chen, L., Ji, H. L., Tse, H. F., Fu, Q.-L., & Lian, Q. (2016). Mesenchymal stem cells and immunomodulation: Current status and future prospects. *Cell Death & Disease*, *7*(1), e2062. PMID: 26794657

Gaowgzeh, R. A. M., & Chevidikunnan, M. F., BinMulayh, E. A., & Khan, F. (2020). Effect of spinal decompression therapy and core stabilization exercises in management of lumbar disc prolapse: A single blind randomized controlled trial. *Journal of Back and Musculoskeletal Rehabilitation*, *33*(2), 225–231. PMID: 31282394

Gao, Y., Wang, Y., Wu, Y., & Liu, S. (2024). Biomaterials targeting the microenvironment for spinal cord injury repair: Progression and perspectives. *Frontiers in Cellular Neuroscience*, *18*, 1362494. PMID: 38784712

García-Jaén, M., Del Barrio-Ventura, A., Sanchis-Soler, G., & Sebastiá-Amat, S. (2025). Exercise-based therapeutic interventions for lumbar disc herniation: A narrative review.

Gautam, D., Vivekanandan, S., & Mazur, M. D. (2025). Robotic spine surgery: Systematic review of common error types and best practices. *Operative Neurosurgery (Hagerstown, Md.)*, *28*(3), 295–302. PMID: 39037253

Gillispie, G., Prim, P., Copus, J., Fisher, J., Mikos, A. G., Yoo, J. J., Atala, A., & Lee, S. J. (2020). Assessment methodologies for extrusion-based bioink printability. *Biofabrication*, *12*(2), 022003. PMID: 31972558

Giraldo, J. P., Cho, S. S., Eghrari, N. B., Dholaria, N., Farber, S. H., Ehredt, R. B., & Uribe, J. S. (2025). Advances in neurosurgical education: Literature review of mixed-reality simulation models and novel mixed-reality spine prototype. *Journal of Neurosurgery. Spine*, *42*(3), 385–398. PMID: 39752650

Girardo, M., Fusini, F., Messina, D., Gargiulo, G., Cinnella, P., Amico, S., & Costa, P. (2025). Comparison of free-hand technique and patient-specific guiding template for pedicle screws positioning in adolescent idiopathic scoliosis surgery using neurophysiological monitoring. *European Spine Journal : Official Publication of the European Spine Society, the European Spinal Deformity Society, and the European Section of the Cervical Spine Research Society*, •••, 1–7. PMID: 40760191

Gudapati, H., Dey, M., & Ozbolat, I. (2019). A comprehensive review on droplet-based bioprinting: Past, present and future. *Biomaterials*, *102*, 20–42. PMID: 27318933

Guo, A. J. X., & Zhu, F. (2019). A CNN-based spatial feature fusion algorithm for hyperspectral imagery classification. *IEEE Transactions on Geoscience and Remote Sensing*, *57*(9), 7170–7181. DOI: 10.1109/TGRS.2019.2911993

Gu, Z., Fu, J., Lin, H., & He, Y. (2020). Development of 3D bioprinting: From printing methods to biomedical applications. *Asian Journal of Pharmaceutical Sciences*, *15*(4), 529–557. PMID: 33193859

Guzzi, G., Ricciuti, R. A., Della Torre, A., Lo Turco, E., Lavano, A., Longhini, F., & La Torre, D. (2024). Intraoperative neurophysiological monitoring in neurosurgery. *Journal of Clinical Medicine*, *13*(10), 2966. PMID: 38792507

Hammond, J., & Priola, S. (2025). Advancements in robotic-assisted spine surgery: A literature review and technology comparison. *Interdisciplinary Neurosurgery : Advanced Techniques and Case Management*, •••, 102056.

Hasan, S., Härtl, R., & Hofstetter, C. P. (2019). The benefit zone of full-endoscopic spine surgery. *Journal of Spine Surgery*, *5*(Suppl 1), S41. PMID: 31380492

Hey, G., Guyot, M., Carter, A., & Lucke-Wold, B. (2023). Augmented reality in neurosurgery: A new paradigm for training. *Medicina*, *59*(10), 1721. PMID: 37893439

Hinojosa González, L. (2023). Evaluación de la morbilidad y mortalidad postoperatoria en el paciente neuroquirúrgico: valor de 2 escalas predictivas.

Hossain, S. F., Al Amin, M., Liza, I. A., Ahmed, S., Haque, M. M., Islam, M. A., & Akter, S. (2023). AI-Based Brain MRI Segmentation for Early Diagnosis and Treatment Planning of Low-Grade Gliomas in the USA. *British Journal of Nursing Studies*, *3*(2), 37–55.

Howard, V. J., & Mcdonnell, M. N. (2015). Physical Activity in Primary Stroke Prevention. *Stroke*, *46*(6), 1735–1739. PMID: 25882053

Huang, M., Tetreault, T. A., Vaishnav, A., York, P. J., & Staub, B. N. (2021). The current state of navigation in robotic spine surgery. *Annals of Translational Medicine*, *9*(1), 86. PMID: 33553379

Hu, Y., Zhang, H., Wei, H., Cheng, H., Cai, J., Chen, X., Xia, L., Wang, H., & Chai, R. (2022). Scaffolds with anisotropic structure for neural tissue engineering. *Engineered Regeneration*, *3*, 154–162.

Iaquinta, M. R., Mazzoni, E., Bononi, I., Rotondo, J. C., Mazziotta, C., & Montesi, M.. (2019). Adult stem cells for bone regeneration and repair. *Frontiers in Cell and Developmental Biology*, *7*, 268. PMID: 31799249

Jahangiri, F. R., Jahangiri, R. H., Asad, H., Farooq, L., Khattak, W. H., Jahangiri, R. H., & Khattak, W. H. (2022). Scoliosis Corrective Surgery With Continuous Intraoperative Neurophysiological Monitoring (IONM). *Cureus, 14*(10). PMID: 36381772

Jain, D. (2019). *Data Preprocessing in Data Mining-GeeksforGeeks* [online]. GeeksforGeeks.

Jena, R., Sethi, D., Chaudhari, P., & Gee, J. (2024). Deep learning in medical image registration: Magic or mirage? *Advances in Neural Information Processing Systems, 37*, 108331–108353.

Jeraj, A. R., & Zameer, Z. (2025). AI-Enhanced Bioactive 3D-Printed Scaffolds for Tissue Regeneration: Innovations in Healing and Functional Additives. *Journal of Computing & Biomedical Informatics, 8*(02).

Jia, Z., & Li, W. (2024). Nanosystems-enabled regenerative strategies for spinal cord injury: Recent advances and future prospects. *Materials & Design, 237*, 112617.

Jiu, J., Liu, H. F., Li, D. J., Li, J. R., Liu, L., Yang, W. J., Yan, L., Li, S. Y., Zhang, J., & Li, X. K.. (2024). 3D bioprinting approaches for spinal cord injury repair. *Biofabrication, 16*(3), 032003. PMID: 38569491

Kapila, R., & Saleti, S. (2024). Federated learning-based disease prediction: A fusion approach with feature selection and extraction. *Biomedical Signal Processing and Control, 100*, 106961. DOI: 10.1016/j.bspc.2024.106961

Kaplan, N., Marques, M., Scharf, I., Yang, K., Alkureishi, L., Purnell, C., & Zhao, L. (2023). Virtual reality and augmented reality in plastic and craniomaxillofacial surgery: A scoping review. *Bioengineering (Basel, Switzerland), 10*(4), 480. PMID: 37106667

Kenkre, J., & Bassett, J. (2018). The bone remodeling cycle. *Annals of Clinical Biochemistry, 55*, 308–327. PMID: 29368538

Kim, H. S., Wu, P. H., & Jang, I. T. (2020). Current and future of endoscopic spine surgery: What are the common procedures we have now and what lies ahead? *World Neurosurgery, 140*, 642–653. PMID: 32797991

Kim, S., & Kim, K. H. (2021). How to use neuronavigation for the brain. *J Korean Soc Ster Func Neuro., 17*(2), 126–132. DOI: 10.52662/jksfn.2021.0008

Kingsly, E. N., Bozkurt, I., & Chaurasia, B. (2023). Neuro-navigation: Equipment, tips, and tricks on brain navigated surgery. *Indian Journal of Neurosurgery, 12*(03), 193–202.

Koch, L., Gruene, M., & Unger, C. (2019). Laser-assisted cell printing. *Current Pharmaceutical Biotechnology, 14*, 91–97. PMID: 23570054

Krauze, A. V., Zhuge, Y., Zhao, R., Tasci, E., & Camphausen, K. (2022). AI-driven image analysis in central nervous system tumors-traditional machine learning, deep learning and hybrid models. *Journal of Biotechnology and Biomedicine, 5*(1), 1. PMID: 35106480

Kumar, H., & Kim, K. (2020). Stereolithography 3D bioprinting. *Methods in Molecular Biology (Clifton, N.J.), 2140*, 93–108. DOI: 10.1007/978-1-0716-0520-0_6 PMID: 32207107

Kumar, P., Ebbens, S., & Zhao, X. (2021). Inkjet printing of mammalian cells—Theory and applications. *Bioprinting (Amsterdam, Netherlands), 23*, e00157.

Kunwar, D. S., Maurya, V. P., Deivasigamani, B., Mishra, R., & Agrawal, A. (2023). Perspective Chapter: Glioblastoma of the Corpus Callosum. *Glioblastoma-Current Evidence*, 39.

Kwon, B., & Moon, A. (2025). Advances in Endoscopic Lumbar Spine Surgery: A Comprehensive Review of the Techniques used for the Treatment of Lumbar Disc Herniations and Spinal Stenosis and Lumbar Spinal Fusion. *The Spine Journal*. PMID: 40578443

Lacroix, M., Khalifé, M., Ferrero, E., Clément, O., Nguyen, C., & Feydy, A. (2023, October). Scoliosis. [). Thieme Medical Publishers, Inc.]. *Seminars in Musculoskeletal Radiology, 27*(05), 529–544. PMID: 37816361

Łajczak, P., Żerdziński, K., Jóźwik, K., Laskowski, M., & Dymek, M. (2024). Enhancing precision and safety in spinal surgery: A comprehensive review of robotic assistance technologies. *World Neurosurgery, 191*, 109–116. PMID: 39151699

Lang, S. K., Gan, Z. C., Wang, Q., Xu, X. H., Li, F. Y., Zhang, J. S., & Chen, X. L. (2025). Development and Application of the Portable Electromagnetic Navigation for Neurosurgery. *Current Medical Science*, •••, 1–12. PMID: 40397298

Lau, K. K. L., Kwan, K. Y. H., & Cheung, J. P. Y. (2025). Sensitivity of intraoperative electrophysiological monitoring for scoliosis correction in identifying postoperative neurological deficits: A retrospective chart review of the Scoliosis Research Society morbidity and mortality database. *BMC Musculoskeletal Disorders*, *26*(1), 186. PMID: 39994650

Ledda, M., Merco, M., Sciortino, A., Scatena, E., Convertino, A., Lisi, A., & Del Gaudio, C. (2022). Biological response to bioinspired microporous 3D-printed scaffolds for bone tissue engineering. *International Journal of Molecular Sciences*, *23*(5383). PMID: 35628195

Lee, J., Kim, Y., & Kim, E. (2024). Data-driven stroke classification utilizing electromyographic muscle features and machine learning techniques. *Applied Sciences (Basel, Switzerland)*, *14*(18), 8430.

Lee, S., Nam, H., Joo, K. M., & Lee, S. H. (2022). Advances in neural stem cell therapy for spinal cord injury: Safety, efficacy, and future perspectives. *Neurospine*, *19*, 946–960. PMID: 36351442

Li, H. M., Zhang, R. J., & Shen, C. L. (2020). Accuracy of pedicle screw placement and clinical outcomes of robot-assisted technique versus conventional freehand technique in spine surgery from nine randomized controlled trials: A meta-analysis. *Spine*, *45*(2), E111–E119. PMID: 31404053

Li, H., Li, C., Wang, J., Yang, A., Ma, Z., Zhang, Z., & Hua, D. (2023). Review on security of federated learning and its application in healthcare. *Future Generation Computer Systems*, *144*, 271–290. DOI: 10.1016/j.future.2023.02.021

Li, J., Fang, Y., Jin, Z., Wang, Y., & Yu, M. (2020). The impact of robot-assisted spine surgeries on clinical outcomes: A systemic review and meta-analysis. *International Journal of Medical Robotics and Computer Assisted Surgery*, *16*(6), 1–14. PMID: 32725898

Li, T., Yan, J., Li, J., Shang, Y., & Tang, X. (2025). Robot-assisted technique versus freehand technique for spine surgery: An umbrella review. *Annals of Medicine*, *57*(1), 2523564. PMID: 40631354

Liu, K.-C., Chen, Y.-C., Hsieh, C.-F., Wang, M.-H., Zhong, M.-X., & Cheng, N.-C. (2024). Scaffold-free 3D culture systems for stem cell-based tissue regeneration. *APL Bioengineering*, *8*, 041501. PMID: 39364211

Liu, S., Yang, H., Chen, D., Xie, Y. Y., Tai, C. X., Wang, L. D., Wang, P., & Wang, B. (2022). Three-dimensional bioprinting sodium alginate/gelatin scaffold combined with neural stem cells and oligodendrocytes markedly promoting nerve regeneration after spinal cord injury. *Regenerative Biomaterials*, *9*, rbac038. PMID: 35801010

Liu, X. Y., Hao, M. M., Chen, Z. J., Zhang, T., Huang, J., Dai, J. W., & Zhang, Z. J. (2021). 3D bioprinted neural tissue constructs for spinal cord injury repair. *Biomaterials*, *272*, 120771. PMID: 33798962

Liu, Y., Wu, J., Zhou, L., Tang, X., Wu, S., & Ji, P. (2025). Research on the combination of algorithms and mixed reality for the localization of perforator vessels in anterolateral thigh and free fibula flaps. *Frontiers in Virtual Reality*, *6*, 1420404.

Liu, Z., Huang, J., Zhang, H., Zhang, S., Dai, H., Jiang, Y., & Shan, Z. (2025). The application of robotic and artificial intelligence technologies in spinal surgery: A review focused on prospects in remote areas of China. *Journal of Robotic Surgery*, *19*(1), 1–17. PMID: 40940589

Lu, D. Z., Yang, Y., Zhang, P. P., Ma, Z. J., Li, W. T., Song, Y., Feng, H. Y., Yu, W. Q., Ren, F. C., & Li, T.. (2022). Development and application of three-dimensional bioprinting scaffold in the repair of spinal cord injury. *Tissue Engineering and Regenerative Medicine*, *19*(5), 1113–1127. PMID: 35767151

MacDonald, J., & Tsirikos, A. I. (2025). The use of neurophysiology in spinal surgery: Who, what, when and how? *Orthopaedics and Trauma*.

MacLean, L., Hersh, A. M., Bhimreddy, M., Jiang, K., Davidar, A. D., Weber-Levine, C., ... & Theodore, N. (2024). Comparison of accuracy, revision, and perioperative outcomes in robot-assisted spine surgeries: systematic review and meta-analysis. *Journal of Neurosurgery: Spine, 1*(aop), 1-13.

Malbert, C. H. (2021). Open-source 3D printable frameless stereotaxic system for young and adult pigs. *Journal of Neuroscience Methods*, *359*, 109222. PMID: 34004201

Malham, G. M., Wells-Quinn, T. A., Nowitzke, A. M., Mobbs, R. J., & Sekhon, L. H. (2024). Challenges in contemporary spinal robotics: Encouraging spine surgeons to drive transformative changes in the development of future robotic platforms. *Journal of Spine Surgery*, *10*(3), 540. PMID: 39399084

Mammen, P. M. (2021, January 14). *Federated learning: Opportunities and challenges.* arXiv.org. https://arxiv.org/abs/2101.05428

Manning, E., & Emerson, R. (2024). Intraoperative monitoring of scoliosis surgery in young patients. *Journal of Clinical Neurophysiology*, *41*(2), 138–147. PMID: 38306222

Masaoka, T., Yoshii, T., Yuasa, M., Yamada, T., Taniyama, T., Torigoe, I., Shinomiya, K., Okawa, A., Morita, S., & Sotome, S. (2016). Bone defect regeneration by a combination of a β-tricalcium phosphate scaffold and bone marrow stromal cells in a non-human primate model. *The Open Biomedical Engineering Journal*, *10*, 2–11. PMID: 27073583

Ma, Y. H., Liang, Q. Y., Ding, Y., Han, I., & Zeng, X. (2022). Multimodal repair of spinal cord injury with mesenchymal stem cells. *Neurospine*, *19*, 616–629. PMID: 36203288

McCracken, D. J., Schupper, A. J., Lakomkin, N., Malcolm, J., Painton Bray, D., & Hadjipanayis, C. G. (2022). Turning on the light for brain tumor surgery: A 5-aminolevulinic acid story. *Neuro-Oncology*, *24*(Supplement_6), S52–S61. PMID: 36322101

Mohan, P. P., & Ramkumar, G. (2025, June). Experimental Analysis of Brain Tumors Identification Methodology Using Artificial Intelligence (AI) Powered Learning Technique. In *2025 International Conference on Emerging Technologies in Engineering Applications (ICETEA)* (pp. 1-6).

Moradi, S., Mahdizadeh, H., Šarić, T., Kim, J., Harati, J., Shahsavarani, H., Greber, B., & Moore, J. B. (2019). Research and therapy with induced pluripotent stem cells (iPSCs): Social, legal, and ethical considerations. *Stem Cell Research & Therapy, 10,* 341. PMID: 31753034

Moshawrab, M., Adda, M., Bouzouane, A., Ibrahim, H., & Raad, A. (2023). Reviewing federated machine learning and its use in diseases prediction. *Sensors (Basel), 23*(4), 2112. DOI: 10.3390/s23042112 PMID: 36850717

Myeroff, C., & Archdeacon, M. (2011). Autogenous bone graft: Donor sites and techniques. *The Journal of Bone and Joint Surgery. American Volume, 93*(23), 2227–2236. PMID: 22159859

Nagarajan, L., Ghosh, S., Dillon, D., Palumbo, L., Woodland, P., Thalayasingam, P., & Lethbridge, M. (2019). Intraoperative neurophysiology monitoring in scoliosis surgery in children. *Clinical Neurophysiology Practice, 4*, 11–17. PMID: 30828671

Naik, A., Smith, A. D., Shaffer, A., Krist, D. T., Moawad, C. M., MacInnis, B. R., & Arnold, P. M. (2022). Evaluating robotic pedicle screw placement against conventional modalities: A systematic review and network meta-analysis. *Neurosurgical Focus, 52*(1), E10. PMID: 34973681

Nayak, S., & Gupta, N. (2024, June). Enhancing Stroke Prediction with Machine Learning in Smart Healthcare Systems. In *2024 15th International Conference on Computing Communication and Networking Technologies (ICCCNT)* (pp. 1-6). IEEE.

Newsome, P. N., Fox, R., King, A. L., Barton, D., Than, N. N., Moore, J., Corbett, C., Townsend, S., Thomas, J., Guo, K., Hull, D., Beard, H. A., Thompson, J., Atkinson, A., Bienek, C., McGowan, N., Guha, N., Campbell, J., Hollyman, D., & Forbes, S. J. (2018). Granulocyte colony-stimulating factor and autologous CD133-positive stem-cell therapy in liver cirrhosis (REALISTIC): An open-label, randomized, controlled phase 2 trial. *The Lancet. Gastroenterology & Hepatology, 3*(1), 25–36. PMID: 29127060

Olexa, J., Chen, C., Rastogi, P., Sansur, C., Rakovec, M., Saadon, J. R., ... & Woodworth, G. F. (2025). Clinical validation of a rapid, markerless, headset-contained augmented reality stereotactic neuronavigation system. *Journal of Neurosurgery, 1*(aop), 1-7.

Ostrom, Q. T., Price, M., Neff, C., Cioffi, G., Waite, K. A., & Kruchko, C.. (2023). CBTRUS statistical report: Primary brain and other central nervous system tumors diagnosed in the United States in 2016–2020. *Neuro-Oncology*, *25*(Supplement_4), iv1–iv99. DOI: 10.1093/neuonc/noad149 PMID: 37793125

Parajuli, S., Gyawali, P., Subedi, P., Bhatta, O. P., Mukhia, R., Sedain, G., & Sharma, M. R. (2022). Neurosurgery as a career choice among recent medical graduates from the institute of medicine, Nepal: A cross-sectional study. *Nepal J. Neurosci.*, *19*(4), 39–42.

Perez, J. R., Kouroupis, D., Li, D. J., Best, T. M., Kaplan, L., & Correa, D. (2018). Tissue engineering and cell-based therapies for fractures and bone defects. *Frontiers in Bioengineering and Biotechnology*, *6*, 105. PMID: 30109228

Persaud, A., Maus, A., Strait, L., & Zhu, D. (2022). 3D bioprinting with live cells. *Engineered Regeneration*, *3*(4), 292–309.

Peters, D. R., Halimi, F., Ozduman, K., Levivier, M., Conti, A., Reyns, N., & Tuleasca, C. (2023). Resection of the contrast-enhancing tumor in diffuse gliomas bordering eloquent areas using electrophysiology and 5-ALA fluorescence: Evaluation of resection rates and neurological outcome—a systematic review and meta-analysis. *Neurosurgical Review*, *46*(1), 185. PMID: 37498398

Pichaivel, M., Anbumani, G., Theivendren, P., & Gopal, M. (2022). *An overview of brain tumor*. IntechOpen.

Pratt, P., Ives, M., Lawton, G., Simmons, J., Radev, N., Spyropoulou, L., & Yang, G. (2018). Through the HoloLens™ looking glass: Augmented reality for extremity reconstruction surgery using 3D vascular models with perforating vessels. *European Radiology Experimental*, *2*(1), 2. PMID: 29708204

Raju, N. (2024). Data-Driven Neurology: Machine Learning Applications In Stroke Forecasting. *International Journal of Data Science and IoT Management System*, *3*(1), 16–19.

Rauniyar, A., Hagos, D. H., Jha, D., Håkegård, J. E., Bagci, U., Rawat, D. B., & Vlassov, V. (2023). Federated learning for medical applications: A taxonomy, current trends, challenges, and future research directions. *IEEE Internet of Things Journal, 11*(5), 7374–7398.

Rebelo, P., Sousa, C. P., Campos, M. T., & Campos, M. (2024). The Value of Intraoperative Neurophysiological Monitoring During Patient Positioning in Spine Surgery: A Preventive Strategy. *Cureus, 16*(11). PMID: 39677176

Reysner, M., Reysner, T., Janusz, P., Kowalski, G., Geisler-Wojciechowska, A., Grochowicka, M., & Wieczorowska-Tobis, K. (2024). The Influence of Anesthesia on Neuromonitoring During Scoliosis Surgery: A Systematic Review. *NeuroSci, 5*(4), 693–712. PMID: 39728681

Riewruja, K., Tanasansomboon, T., Yingsakmongkol, W., Kotheeranurak, V., Limthongkul, W., Chokesuwattanaskul, R., & Singhatanadgige, W. (2024). A Network Meta-Analysis Comparing the Efficacy and Safety of Pedicle Screw Placement Techniques Using Intraoperative Conventional, Navigation, Robot-Assisted, and Augmented Reality Guiding Systems. *The International Journal of Spine Surgery, 18*(5), 551–570. PMID: 39079746

Rogers, C. M., Jones, P. S., & Weinberg, J. S. (2021). Intraoperative MRI for brain tumors. *Journal of Neuro-Oncology, 151*(3), 479–490. PMID: 33611714

Ruggiero, F. (2024). Application of augmented reality in craniofacial surgery: a feasibility study.

Ruggiero, F., Cercenelli, L., Emiliani, N., Badiali, G., Bevini, M., Zucchelli, M., & Tarsitano, A. (2023). Preclinical application of augmented reality in pediatric craniofacial surgery: An accuracy study. *Journal of Clinical Medicine, 12*(7), 2693. PMID: 37048777

Saini, G., Segaran, N., Mayer, J. L., Saini, A., Albadawi, H., & Oklu, R. (2021). Applications of 3D bioprinting in tissue engineering and regenerative medicine. *Journal of Clinical Medicine, 10*(4966). PMID: 34768485

Salleh, M. I. M., Abdullah, R., & Zakaria, N. (2021). Evaluating the effects of electronic health records system adoption on the performance of Malaysian health care providers. *BMC Medical Informatics and Decision Making, 21*(1), 75. PMID: 33632216

Samprón, N., Lafuente, J., Presa-Alonso, J., Ivanov, M., Hartl, R., & Ringel, F. (2025). Advancing spine surgery: Evaluating the potential for full robotic automation. *Brain & Spine*, •••, 104232. PMID: 40191588

Schneider, D., Brown, E. D., Elsamadicy, A. A., Sciubba, D. M., & Lo, S. F. L. (2025). The Hidden Cost of Robotic Spine Surgery: Real-World Adverse Events Cause 58-Minute Delays and Undermine Economic Viability. *The Spine Journal*.

Schulze, P., O'Connor, C., Anand, N., & Wynne, P. (2020). A rare cause of acute back pain in a young adult: Case report and discussion of calcific discitis. *Journal of Radiology Case Reports*, *14*(10), 1. PMID: 33708337

Shahin, M., Siavashpour, Z., & Beigi, M. (2025). Overview of Radiotherapy Techniques. *From Radiobiology to Radiation Oncology*, 117.

Sharma, N., Mallela, A. N., Khan, T., Canton, S. P., Kass, N. M., Steuer, F., & Andrews, E. G. (2024). Evolution of the meta-neurosurgeon: A systematic review of the current technical capabilities, limitations, and applications of augmented reality in neurosurgery. *Surgical Neurology International*, *15*, 146. PMID: 38742013

Shashidhar, K. (2025). Deep learning-based automated detection of brain tumors using MRI scans and 3d convolutional neural networks. *American Journal of Management and IOT Medical Computing*, *4*(4), 95–102.

Shen, G., Fu, Z., Gui, Y., Susilo, W., & Zhang, M. (2023). Efficient and privacy-preserving online diagnosis scheme based on federated learning in e-healthcare system. *Information Sciences*, *647*, 119261. DOI: 10.1016/j.ins.2023.119261

Shi, Y., Deng, X., Tong, Y., Li, R., Zhang, Y., Ren, L., & Si, W. (2022). Synergistic digital twin and holographic augmented-reality-guided percutaneous puncture of respiratory liver tumor. *IEEE Transactions on Human-Machine Systems*, *52*(6), 1364–1374.

Siapati, E. K., Roubelakis, M. G., & Vassilopoulos, G. (2022). Liver regeneration by hematopoietic stem cells: Have we reached the end of the road? *Cells*, *11*(15), 2312. PMID: 35954155

Singh, M. S., Thongam, K., Choudhary, P., & Bhagat, P. K. (2025). Stroke Risk Prediction and Prevention: Traditional versus Machine Learning Approaches. *Archives of Computational Methods in Engineering*, •••, 1–52.

Singh, V., Malik, M., Kaur, J., Kulandaivelan, S., & Punia, S. (2021). A systematic review and meta-analysis on the efficacy of physiotherapy intervention in management of lumbar prolapsed intervertebral disc. *International Journal of Health Sciences*, *15*(2), 49. PMID: 33708044

Soomro, N. A., Hashimoto, D. A., Porteous, A. J., Ridley, C. J. A., Marsh, W. J., Ditto, R., & Roy, S. (2020). Systematic review of learning curves in robot-assisted surgery. *BJS Open*, *4*(1), 27–44. PMID: 32011823

Spahr, L., Chalandon, Y., Terraz, S., Kindler, V., Rubbia-Brandt, L., Frossard, J. L., Breguet, R., Lanthier, N., Farina, A., Passweg, J., Becker, C. D., & Hadengue, A. (2013). Autologous bone marrow mononuclear cell transplantation in patients with decompensated alcoholic liver disease: A randomized controlled trial. *PLoS One*, *8*(1), e53719. PMID: 23341981

Sridhar, A. N., Briggs, T. P., Kelly, J. D., & Nathan, S. (2017). Training in robotic surgery—An overview. *Current Urology Reports*, *18*(8), 58. PMID: 28647793

Sukho, P., Cohen, A., Hesselink, J. W., Kirpensteijn, J., Verseijden, F., & Bastiaansen-Jenniskens, Y. M. (2018). Adipose tissue-derived stem cell sheet application for tissue healing in vivo: A systematic review. *Tissue Engineering. Part B, Reviews*, *24*(1), 37–52. PMID: 28665192

Sulangi, A. J., Husain, A., Lei, H., & Okun, J. (2024). Neuronavigation in glioma resection: Current applications, challenges, and clinical outcomes. *Frontiers in Surgery*, *11*, 1430567. PMID: 39165667

Sulangi, A. J., Husain, A., Lei, H., & Okun, J. (2025). Neuronavigation in glioma resection: Current applications, challenges, and clinical. *Training and Education in Neurosurgery: Strategies and Challenges for the Next Ten Years*, *II*, 54.

Sung, W. S., Goo, B. H., Kim, E. J., Nam, D. W., Kim, T. H., Park, Y. C., & Seo, B. K. (2020). Efficacy and safety of thread-embedding acupuncture for lumbar herniated intervertebral disc: A systematic review and meta-analysis. *European Journal of Integrative Medicine*, *39*, 101195.

Sun, W. X., Huang, W. Q., Li, H. Y., Wang, H. S., Guo, S. L., Dong, J., & Lin, Y. P. (2023). Clinical efficacy of robotic spine surgery: An updated systematic review of 20 randomized controlled trials. *EFORT Open Reviews*, *8*(11), 841–853. PMID: 37909700

Susskind, R. (2025). *How to Think about AI: A Guide for the Perplexed.* Oxford University Press.

Szymoniuk, M., Mazurek, M., Dryla, A., & Kamieniak, P. (2023). The application of 3D-bioprinted scaffolds for neuronal regeneration after traumatic spinal cord injury—A systematic review of preclinical in vivo studies. *Experimental Neurology*, *363*, 114366. PMID: 36858280

Taghian, A., Abo-Zahhad, M., Sayed, M. S., & Abd El-Malek, A. H. (2023). Virtual and augmented reality in biomedical engineering. *Biomedical Engineering Online*, *22*(1), 76. PMID: 37525193

Tarawneh, A. M., & Salem, K. M. (2021). A systematic review and meta-analysis of randomized controlled trials comparing the accuracy and clinical outcome of pedicle screw placement using robot-assisted technology and conventional freehand technique. *Global Spine Journal*, *11*(4), 575–586. PMID: 32677515

Thakre, G., Raut, R., Puri, C., & Verma, P. (2025). A hybrid deep learning approach for improved detection and prediction of brain stroke. *Applied Sciences (Basel, Switzerland)*, *15*(9), 4639.

Thavarajasingam, S. G., Salih, A., Arif, A., Varadpande, M., Sabeshan, P., Ponniah, H. S., & Ringel, F. (2025). Indications for Surgery Versus Conservative Treatment in The Management of Lumbar Disc Herniations: A Systematic Review. *Brain & Spine*, •••, 105619. PMID: 41078967

Türkkan, A., & Bekar, A. (2024). Evaluation of the Use of Intraoperative Neuronavigation in the Surgery of Brain Tumors: Single Center Experience and Retrospective Analysis of 172 Cases. *Uludağ Üniversitesi Tıp Fakültesi Dergisi*, *50*(2), 289–297.

Usharani, S., Bala, P. M., kumar, T. A., & Selvam, G. G. (2025). Automated 3D U-Net Framework for Brain Tumor Segmentation and Classification with Insights Into AI-Driven Cancer Research Applications. *Targeted Chemotherapy with Personalized Immunotherapy: An AI Approach*, 279-307.

Vadalà, G., De Salvatore, S., Ambrosio, L., Russo, F., Papalia, R., & Denaro, V. (2020). Robotic spine surgery and augmented reality systems: A state of the art. *Neurospine*, *17*(1), 88. PMID: 32252158

Ventura, R. D. (2021). An overview of laser-assisted bioprinting (LAB) in tissue engineering applications. *Medical Lasers*, *10*, 76–81. DOI: 10.25289/ML.2021.10.2.76

Viglialoro, R. M., Condino, S., Turini, G., Carbone, M., Ferrari, V., & Gesi, M. (2021). Augmented reality, mixed reality, and hybrid approach in healthcare simulation: A systematic review. *Applied Sciences (Basel, Switzerland)*, *11*(5), 2338.

Wang, X., Yang, J., Zhou, B., Tang, L., & Liang, Y. (2025). Integrating Mixed Reality, Augmented Reality, and Artificial Intelligence in Complex Liver Surgeries: Enhancing Precision, Safety, and Outcomes. *iLIVER*, 100167.

Wang, W., & Yeung, K. W. K. (2017). Bone grafts and biomaterials substitutes for bone defect repair: A review. *Bioactive Materials*, *2*, 224–247. PMID: 29744432

Wang, Y., Xiao, Y., Wang, J., Rexiti, P., & Wang, Y. (2025). Spine-specific robots may offer superior screw placement accuracy in spinal surgery procedures. A systematic review and network and proportional meta-analysis. *Journal of Orthopaedic Surgery and Research*, *20*(1), 1–23. PMID: 41137102

World Health Organization. *WHO.(2024, August 7). The top 10 causes of death.*

Wu, P. H., Kim, H. S., & Jang, I. T. (2020). A narrative review of development of full-endoscopic lumbar spine surgery. *Neurospine*, *17*(Suppl 1), S20. PMID: 32746515

Xie, Z., Gao, M., Lobo, A. O., & Webster, T. J. (2020). 3D bioprinting in tissue engineering for medical applications: The classic and the hybrid. *Polymers, 12*(1717).

Yang, V. (2015). Recent advance in visible spectrum surgical navigation. CLEO: 2015.

Ye, D., Wang, Q., Yang, Y., Chen, B., Zhang, F., Wang, Z., & Luan, Z. (2023). Identifying genes that affect differentiation of human neural stem cells and myelination of mature oligodendrocytes. *Cellular and Molecular Neurobiology*, *43*, 2337–2358. PMID: 36547781

Yuan, T. Y., Zhang, J., Yu, T., Wu, J. P., & Liu, Q. Y. (2022). 3D bioprinting for spinal cord injury repair. *Frontiers in Bioengineering and Biotechnology*, *10*, 847344. PMID: 35519617

Yunus, S. N., Chong, H. N., Lee, Z. Y., Osman, R., Goh, K. J., Chiu, C. K., & Hasan, M. S. (2025). Association of perioperative intravenous lignocaine and intraoperative neuromonitoring in adolescent idiopathic scoliosis surgery: A retrospective study. *Perioperative Medicine (London, England)*, *14*(1), 1–10. PMID: 40616131

Zarepour, A., Hooshmand, S., Gokmen, A., Zarrabi, A., & Mostafavi, E. (2021). Spinal cord injury management through the combination of stem cells and implantable 3D bioprinted platforms. *Cells*, *10*(3189). PMID: 34831412

Zhang, B., Shi, H., & Wang, H. (2023). Machine learning and AI in cancer prognosis, prediction, and treatment selection: A critical approach. *Journal of Multidisciplinary Healthcare*, *16*, 1779–1791. DOI: 10.2147/JMDH.S410301 PMID: 37398894

Zhang, D., Cui, X., Zheng, J., Zhang, S., Wang, M., Lu, W., Sang, L., & Li, W. (2021). Neurosurgical robot-assistant stereoelectroencephalography system: Operability and accuracy. *Brain and Behavior*, *11*(10), e2347. PMID: 34520631

Zhang, J., Yang, P., Zeng, L., Li, S., & Zhou, J. (2024). Ventilator-associated pneumonia prediction models based on AI: Scoping review. *JMIR Medical Informatics*, *12*, e57026. DOI: 10.2196/57026 PMID: 38771220

Zhang, W. C., Zheng, M. L., Liu, J., Jin, F., Dong, X. Z., Guo, M., & Li, T. (2021). Modulation of cell behavior by 3D biocompatible hydrogel microscaffolds with precise configuration. *Nanomaterials (Basel, Switzerland), 11*(9), 2325. PMID: 34578641

Zhao, Y., Jia, Z., Aili, A., & Muheremu, A. (2025). Mechanisms and management of self-resolving lumbar disc herniation: Bridging molecular pathways to non-surgical clinical success. *Journal of Orthopaedic Surgery and Research, 20*(1), 528. PMID: 40426259

Zheng, Y., Gallegos, C. M., Xue, H., Li, S., Kim, D. H., Zhou, H., Xia, X., Liu, Y., & Cao, Q. (2022). Transplantation of human induced pluripotent stem cell-derived neural progenitor cells promotes forelimb functional recovery after cervical spinal cord injury. *Cells, 11*, 2765. PMID: 36078173

Zhou, D., Li, X., Wei, S., Yu, C., Wang, D., Li, Y., & Zhang, X. Y. (2024). Transcranial direct current stimulation combined with repetitive transcranial magnetic stimulation for depression: A randomized clinical trial. *JAMA Network Open, 7*(11), e2444306–e2444306. PMID: 39535797

Zubair Rahman, A. M. J., Gupta, M., Aarathi, S., Mahesh, T. R., Vinoth Kumar, V., Yogesh Kumaran, S., & Guluwadi, S. (2024). Advanced AI-driven approach for enhanced brain tumor detection from MRI images utilizing EfficientNetB2 with equalization and homomorphic filtering. *BMC Medical Informatics and Decision Making, 24*(1), 113. PMID: 38689289

About the Contributors

Soobia Saeed is working at Taylors University, Malaysia. Previously, she was a Director of ORIC at Sohail University formerly Jinnah Medical and Dental College (JMDC) and Assistant professor in Sohail university as well. She was leading an ethical review committee in JMDC and led many other industrial projects and pharmaceutical projects. She has experience in pharmaceutical collaboration as well. She did Ph. D in computing engineering from Universiti Teknologi Malaysia (UTM), Malaysia. Her PhD thesis is relevant to Artificial intelligence in healthcare. Her research interest in neurosurgery, oncology, neurosciences, and artificial intelligence encapsulating 90 impactful articles that contribute to the frontiers of knowledge in machine learning, artificial intelligence, computational neuroscience, bioinformatics and computing, and ubiquitous computing. This comprehensive body of work reflects her commitment to advancing the understanding and application of cutting-edge technologies to address contemporary challenges. The bulk of her contributions lie in machine learning, computational neurosciences, and artificial intelligence, where she has explored innovative approaches to address complex problems. These articles, published in journals indexed in the Emerging Sources Citation Index (ESCI), Science Citation Index (SCI), highlighting the clinical relevance and impact of my research in the medical domain and Institute for Scientific Information (ISI), underscoring the significance of her work in shaping the future computational neuroscience and other medical diseases solved by artificial intelligence.

Mohsin Qadeer is an Associate Professor at Agha Khan University Hospital and Medicare Cardiac and General Hospital (MGCH). He is one of the best neurosurgeons in Karachi, with a high patient satisfaction rate. He completed his MBBS and FCPS from Karachi, Pakistan. He completed his house job at Liaquat National Hospital as a house officer and resident neurosurgeon. He has an expert specialization in neurosurgery, which involves surgical treatment of neurological conditions such as peripheral nerve injury, spinal arthritis, cerebrospinal fluid leakage, brain tumors, etc. He has many publications, including national and international publications. Dr. Mohsin Qadeer has authored over 21 impactful articles. Dr. Mohsin Qadeer is associated with renowned hospitals, including Medicare Cardiac and General Hospital (MGCH), the National Medical Complex (NMC), Agha Khan Hospital University, and Ziauddin Hospital. He continued serving in different neurosurgery departments for years, treating all kinds of neurological conditions. A neurosurgeon also specializes in providing pre- and post-surgical care to patients. While working in neurosurgery, he focuses on the treatment of neurological conditions by using surgical methods. His exposure throughout the years of professional practice resulted in the enrichment of treatment skills across the vast field of neurosurgery. He has also been working on risk assessment of neurological conditions as well as their prevention and management. Based on existing conditions, he provides customized treatment plans for patients of all age groups. His expertise in advanced neurosurgery makes him one of the top certified neurosurgeons in Karachi. Currently he supervises many neurosurgeon residents in MGCH and Agha Khan University Hospital, where he contributes to research work in the neurosurgery field.

***

Muhammad Bilal Ashraf is a bioinformatics and data science professional passionate about applying computational methods to healthcare and biomedical research. Currently, I contribute to two research groups at Charité – Universitätsmedizin Berlin: Biosignal Analyst (CCCTIM): Focusing on biological data analysis, signal processing, and integrating traditional and integrative medicine insights into modern healthcare. Machine Learning Researcher (IMI): Developing and applying AI methods for medical imaging and healthcare data, with an emphasis on clinical decision support and translational research. Alongside my professional work, I am pursuing a Master's in Bioinformatics at Freie Universität Berlin, where I continue to deepen my expertise in computational biology, genomics, and medical AI. My research background also includes contributing to robotics and AI projects at the Bundesanstalt für Materialforschung und -prüfung (BAM). My core competencies include: Biosignal & Biological Data Analysis Machine Learning & Medical Imaging Bioinformatics Tools & Genomic Data Analysis Translating Complex Healthcare Data into Actionable Insights I am motivated by the intersection of data science, medicine, and bioinformatics, with the goal of advancing patient care and biomedical innovation through AI-driven research.

Ravikumar R. Natarajan is an experienced academician with over 12+ years of teaching and research expertise across institutions in India, the UAE, and the Maldives. He currently serves as an Assistant Professor at Marwadi University, Rajkot, specializing in Machine Learning, Recommender Systems, and AI-driven applications in healthcare and security. He holds a Ph.D. in Machine Learning and Recommender Systems from Amity University, Jaipur, a Master of Engineering in CSE from VMRF University, Salem, and a Bachelor of Engineering in CSE from Anna University. He also has a MiniMBA from the Swiss eLearning Institute. Dr. Ravikumar has authored more than 8+ multiple SCIE/Scopus-indexed journal articles, 25+ IEEE/Springer conference papers, and co-authored a book on Artificial Intelligence. He has also published 9 patents and contributed 10+ book chapters in emerging domains such as Federated Learning, Blockchain, and Digital Twins for IGI Global, Wiley and Springer publisher. He actively mentors students through initiatives like the Research Activities Club (RAC) and Student Research Internship Training (SRIT), promoting innovation and research culture.

Aarthi S is a dedicated Assistant Professor in Computer Science with over six years of teaching experience. She is currently pursuing her Ph.D. at Marwadi University, Gujarat, and holds an M.Phil. and MCA from Bharathiar University, Tamil Nadu. Throughout her academic career, Aarthi has specialized in programming languages such as C++, Java, and C, and contributed to research in recommender systems and AI-related data privacy. She has published journal articles, contributed to book chapters, and actively participated in technical workshops. Known for her student mentorship and engagement in academic events, Aarthi remains committed to fostering innovation and excellence in computer science education.

Shreha S. A. is associated with the field of Clinical Psychology at PSG College of Arts and Science, Coimbatore, India. Her academic interests focus on understanding psychological processes, mental health assessment, and therapeutic interventions across diverse populations. She is engaged in developing a strong foundation in evidence-based clinical practices, psychological evaluation, and applied research methods. Through her academic training, she demonstrates a commitment to ethical practice, professional competence, and the promotion of mental well-being, with an emphasis on integrating psychological theory with real-world clinical applications.

Lee Seonghyeok is an undergraduate student in the Bachelor of Information Technology (Software Engineering) program at Taylor's University, Malaysia. His research interests include artificial intelligence, federated learning, and privacy-preserving data systems, with a particular focus on healthcare and medical technology applications. He has participated in multidisciplinary projects exploring AI-driven disease prediction and smart healthcare solutions.

Index

A

B

D

I

L

M

N

R

www.ingramcontent.com/pod-product-compliance
Lightning Source LLC
LaVergne TN
LVHW080855300926
849162LV00003B/428
9798337362342